Mediterranean Diet

The Best Mediterranean Recipes to Lose Weight

Jessica Moore

Table of Contents

thought of as universal. As befitting its nature, it is presented without assurance regarding its prolonged validity or interim quality. Trademarks that are mentioned are done without written consent and can in no way be considered an endorsement from the trademark holder.

Introduction

Congratulations and thank you so much for purchasing *Mediterranean Diet*!

If you have been on the hunt for a different type of diet that can actually help you achieve your weight loss goals while consuming delicious food, you have come to the right place to start your journey!

The Mediterranean Diet is unlike any other, especially in the way that there are no hard set of rules to follow. Why? Because there is no "right" method to do this diet! It's actually based on the way folks ate back in the sixties in the beautiful countries of Greece and Italy. Health during this decade was outstanding, thanks to the traditional foods these people consumed.

Consider the following information as a good guideline to follow if you want to lose weight in the Mediterranean Diet:

Focus on eating seafood, fish, spices, herbs, bread, whole grains, potatoes, legumes, seeds, nuts, fruits, and veggies.

You can also consume yogurt, eggs, cheese, and poultry in moderation.

Only consume red meat on ***rare occasions***.

And do your best to avoid foods that are highly processed, refined oils and grains, processed meats, added sugars, and overly sweetened beverages.

- Hot dogs, sausages, etc.
- Canola oil, soybean oil, etc.
- Trans fats in margarine

- Pasta, white bread, and other refined wheat products
- Sugar, ice cream, candy, soda, etc.

Basically, the Mediterranean diet is one that highly promotes consuming plant foods and avoiding animal products. But don't leave out the seafood and fish!

That being said, the pages of this book are packed with easy to make delicious recipes that your entire family will enjoy! From breakfast to dessert, there are a plethora of Mediterranean recipes for any occasion!

While there are tons of books out there regarding the Mediterranean Diet, this one, in particular, focuses on quality recipes that you can make right at home! Instead of surfing the web for recipes, you have 50+ to get you started on the right foot on the Mediterranean train to fuel your weight loss journey!

Breakfast Recipes

Spinach, Tomato, and Feta Scrambled Eggs

What's in it:

- Pepper and salt
- 2 tbsp. cubed feta cheese
- 3 eggs
- 1 C. baby spinach leaves
- 1/3 C. tomato
- 1 tbsp. vegetable oil

How it's made:

- Warm oil. Sauté spinach and tomato together in oil till spinach wilts.
- Pour eggs into the pan. Mix well.
- After about 30 seconds, mix in feta cheese.
- Cook till eggs are done to your liking.
- Season with pepper and salt as needed.

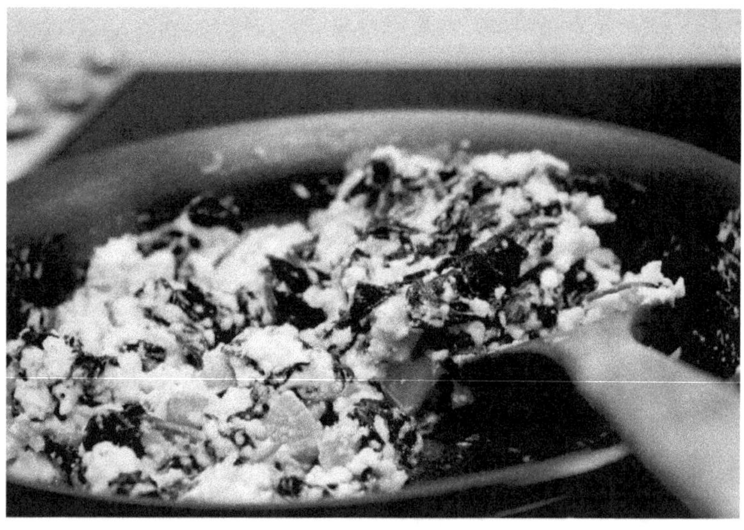

Avocado Toast with Fried Egg

What's in it:

- Pepper and salt
- ¼ tsp. cayenne pepper
- 1 sliced tomato
- Alfalfa sprouts
- 2 eggs
- ½ tsp. olive oil
- 2 slices toasted bread
- 1 avocado

How it's made:

- Cut and dice avocado. Place in bowl. Add cayenne pepper and olive oil to avocado and with a fork, mash.
- Toast bread.
- Slice tomato.
- Fry egg the way you like. (I like sunny-side up best!)
- Spread avocado mixture onto toast. Then top with sliced tomato and alfalfa sprouts.
- Place fried egg on top of sprouts.
- Season with pepper, salt, and spices if desired.

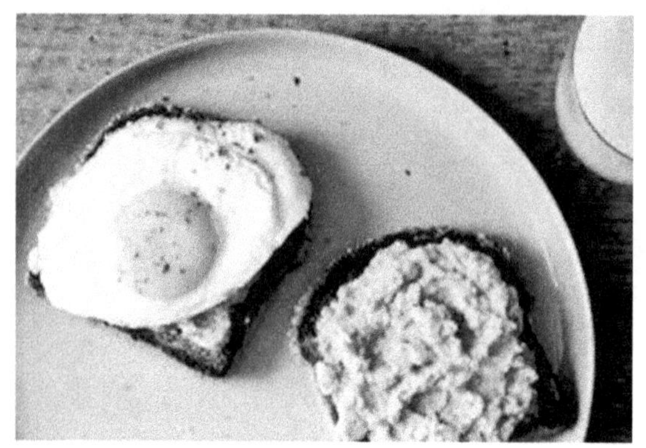

Mediterranean Omelet

What's in it:

- 1 tbsp. romesco sauce
- 1 tbsp. crumbled feta cheese
- 1 quartered artichoke heart
- 2 tbsp. sliced olives
- 2 tbsp. diced tomato
- Pepper and salt
- Oregano
- 1 tbsp. cream
- 2 eggs
- 1 tbsp. oil

How it's made:

- Warm up oil. Add pepper, salt, oregano, cream, and eggs to pain.
- Cook egg mixture till it just begins to set, then add artichoke, feta cheese, olives, and tomatoes.
- Fold half of egg mixture over the other and continue cooking till set.
- Top with romesco sauce when serving! Enjoy!

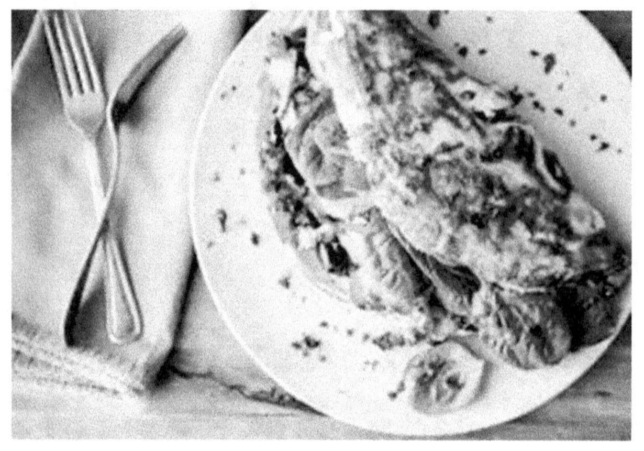

Peaches and Cream

What's in it:

- Sprinkle of caster sugar
- Fresh thyme
- Pistachios or almonds
- Honey
- Crumbled ricotta cheese
- 1 peach or nectarine per person

How it's made:

- Wash and dry peaches. Cut in half and take out stones.
- Sprinkle peaches with caster sugar upon the cut sides.
- Preheat griddle or a grill. Add peaches and sear till just softened.
- Serve warm with a dollop of ricotta, topped with a drizzle of honey, nuts, and sprigs of thyme.

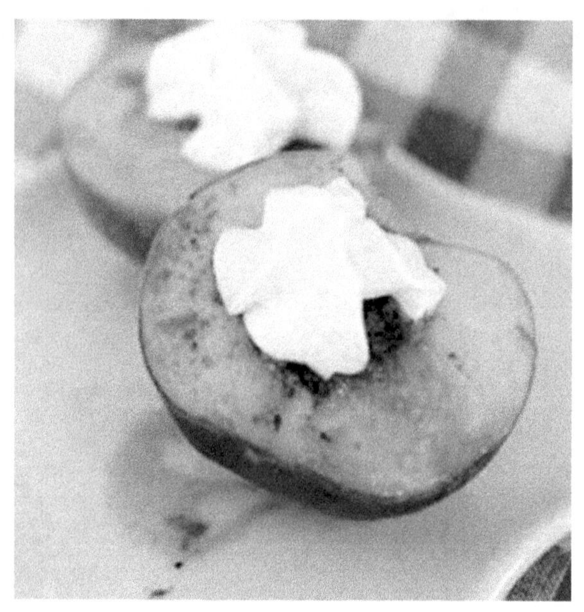

Greek Style Scrambled Eggs

What's in it:

- Pepper and salt
- 1 tsp. mint
- 1-2 tsp. oregano
- 1 tbsp. crumbled feta cheese
- 2 eggs
- 1 tbsp. tomato paste combined with 2-3 tbsp. water
- 10 ounces halved cherry tomatoes
- 1 minced clove of garlic
- 1 chopped onion
- Olive oil

How it's made:

- Warm up olive oil. Sauté onion until softened. Then add garlic and sauté 60 seconds. Place tomatoes in the pan and sauté 2 more minutes.
- Mix water with tomato paste. Add it to the pan and allow to simmer 5-7 minutes till tomatoes become wilted.
- Beat eggs and pour into pan. Heat 2 minutes till they start to thicken.
- Take mixture from pan and transfer to serving plate.
- Season with salt and sprinkle with feta cheese, mint, and oregano. Enjoy!

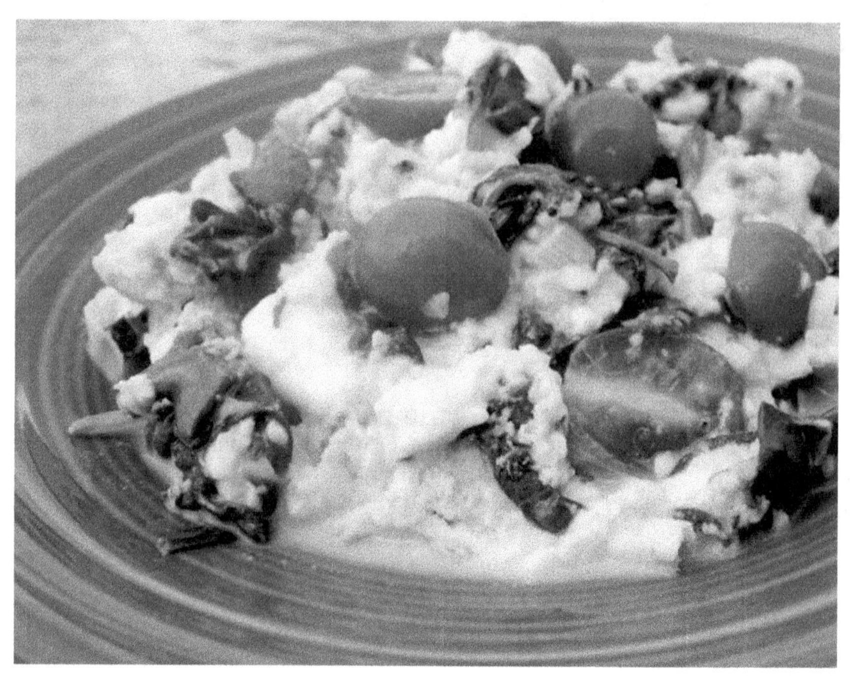

Tahini Feta Toast

What's in it:

- Pepper
- 2 tsp. pine nuts
- 2 tsp. crumbled feta cheese
- 1 tsp. water
- Juice of ½ a lemon
- 1 tbsp. tahini
- 2 slices whole wheat bread

How it's made:

- Combine lemon juice with water and tahini. The mixture should be a bit thinner than peanut butter. If too thick, add a bit more water.
- Toast bread.
- Spread a nice thick layer of tahini mixture onto toast. Sprinkle with a bit of pepper, along with pine nuts and feta cheese.

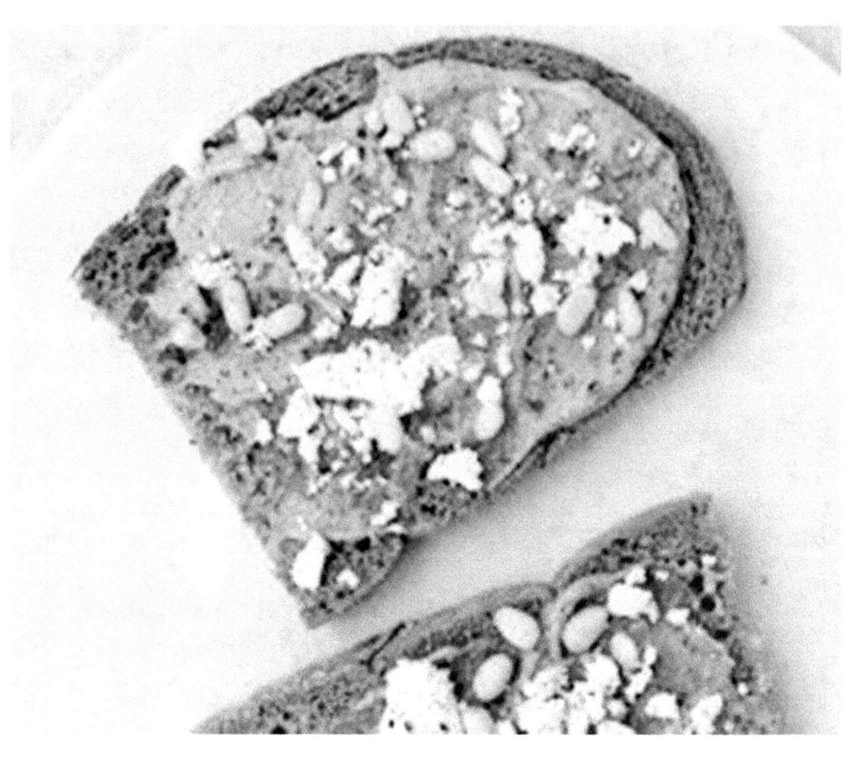

Whole Wheat Olive and Feta Cheese Bread

What's in it:

- 1 C. + 2 tbsp. warm water
- ½ C. crumbled feta cheese
- 1 – 1 ½ C. chopped olive
- 2-3 tbsp. oregano
- ¼ C. olive oil
- 2 tsp. instant dry yeast
- 2 C. all-purpose flour
- 2 C. whole wheat flour

How it's made:

- Combine water with flours and yeast. Add olive oil and salt, incorporate well.
- On a floured surface, turn out the dough. Stretch away from you and roll it back. Do this till dough is smooth and elastic, about 7-10 minutes.
- Roll dough into a ball and place in a bowl covered with plastic wrap. Let sit at room temp for 1 hour.
- Split dough into 2 balls. Stretch each out to form a long piece of dough.
- Add half of oregano, feta, and olives to both halves.
- Put balls of dough onto a pan and slightly flatten. Let sit half an hour.
- Ensure oven is preheated to 425 degrees.
- Sprinkle flour over each piece of dough and make a slit in each.
- Bake 30 minutes. Bread will be slightly moist. Allow to cool before devouring!

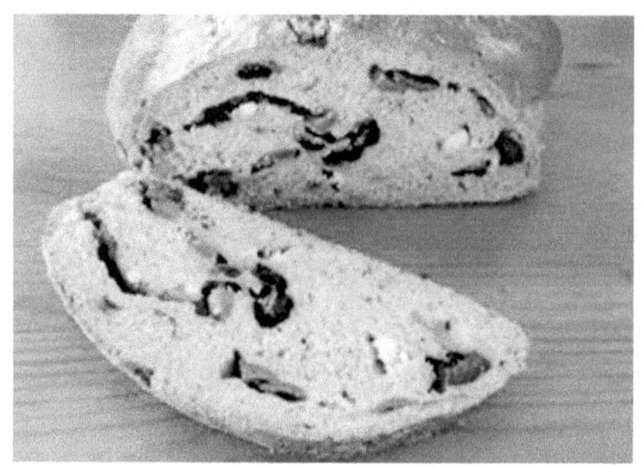

Mediterranean Muffins

What's in it:

Dry Components:

- 2 tsp. orange zest
- ½ tsp. baking soda
- 1 tsp. baking powder
- ½ tsp. salt
- 1/3 C. sugar
- 1 C. whole wheat pastry flour
- 1 C. oats

Wet Components:

- 1 C. blueberries
- ¼ C. chopped dates
- ¾ C. chopped toasted pecans
- ¼ C. boiling water
- ¾ C. natural applesauce
- 1 beaten eggs
- 1 ¼ tsp. vanilla extract
- 1 C. low-fat buttermilk

How it's made:

- Ensure oven is preheated to 375 degrees. Grease a muffin tin liberally.
- Mix together all dry components till combined.
- Mix together all wet components till combined.
- Add wet and dry mixtures together, stirring till well incorporated.
- Fold in nuts, blueberries, and dates.

- Lastly, mix in boiling water. Allow mixture to sit untouched 15 minutes.
- Pour batter into muffin tin. Bake 20-22 minutes.
- Let cool before eating.

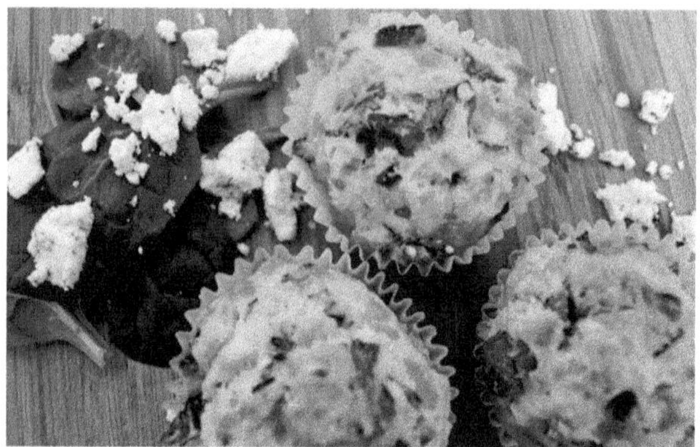

Breakfast Egg Muffins

What's in it:

- Pepper and salt
- 1 chopped tomatoes
- ¼ chopped red pepper
- 4 tbsp. parmesan cheese
- 2 tbsp. skim milk
- 3 eggs
- ¼ C. chopped leek
- ¼ C. chopped baby spinach
- ¼ C. low-fat shredded cheddar cheese

How it's made:

- Ensure oven is preheated to 375 degrees. Grease a muffin tin.
- Whisk Parmesan cheese, milk, and eggs together. Season with pepper and salt.
- Stir in veggies.
- Pour mixture into muffin tin.
- Split up cheddar cheese among muffins.
- Bake 15-20 minutes.

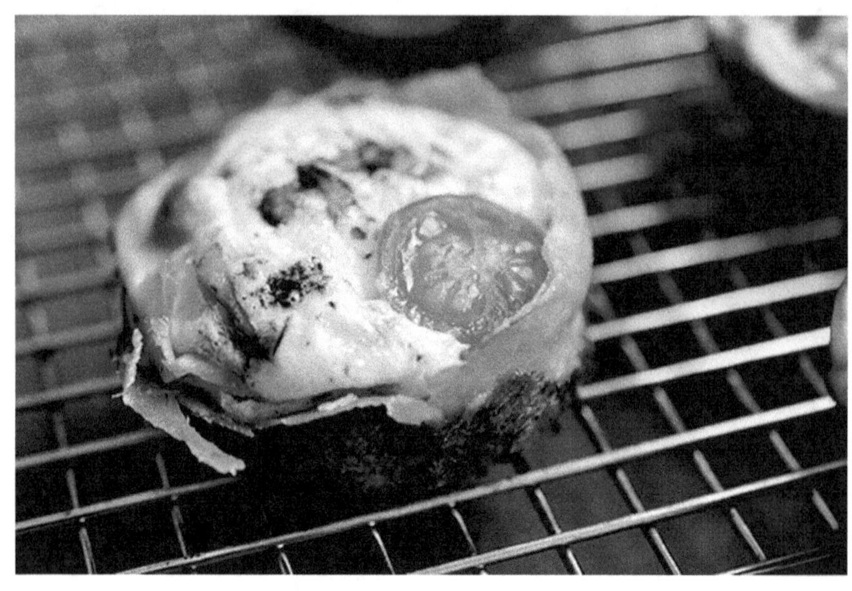

Baked Spinach and Eggs

What's in it:

- 1 tbsp. crumbled feta cheese
- Pepper and salt
- 4 eggs
- 6 C. baby spinach

How it's made:

- Ensure oven is preheated to 400 degrees. Grease ramekins.
- Put spinach in a skillet and add 2-3 tbsp. water. Cook 3-4 minutes until wilted.
- Drain water. Split up spinach leaves evenly between ramekins.
- Crack eggs over spinach. Season with pepper and salt.
- Sprinkle with feta cheese.
- Bake 15-18 minutes till eggs are cooked.

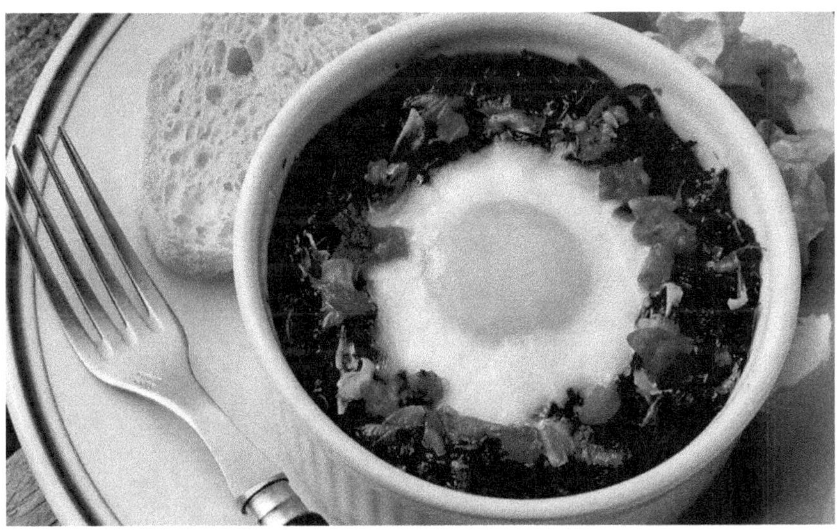

Lunch Recipes

Mediterranean Power Bowl

What's in it:

- ½ C. crumbled feta cheese
- Chopped parsley
- 1 tsp. oregano
- 1 tsp. dill
- 2 minced cloves garlic
- 1 C. halved grape tomatoes
- 1 chopped cucumber
- 1 can rinsed/drained garbanzo beans
- Chopped romaine
- Cooked quinoa

Dressing:

- ¼ tsp. pepper
- ¼ tsp. salt
- 1 tsp. agave
- 3 tbsp. olive oil
- ¼ C. balsamic vinegar
- Juice of 1 lemon

How it's made:

- Prepare quinoa and set to the side.
- Combine oregano, dill, garlic, tomato, cucumber, and garbanzo beans together.
- Whip up dressing components together. Add to bean mixture.
- When ready to serve, toss romaine, a scoop of quinoa, and a heaping portion of garbanzo bean salad

together. Season with pepper and salt. Top with feta
cheese.

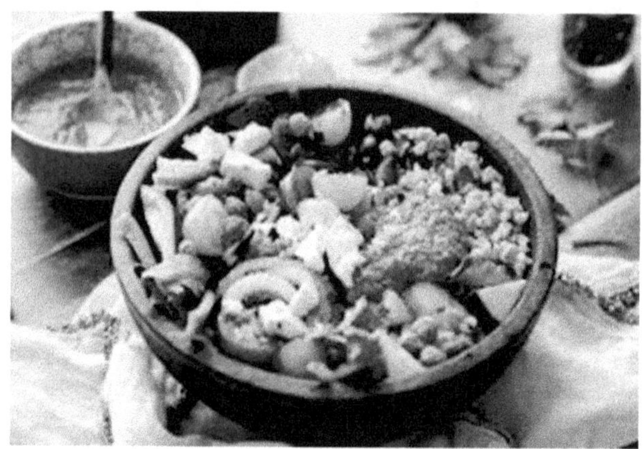

Caprese Style Portobello Mushrooms

What's in it:

- Halved cherry tomatoes
- Portobello mushroom caps
- Shredded mozzarella cheese
- Fresh basil
- Olive oil

How it's made:

- Ensure oven is preheated to 400 degrees. With foil, line a tray.
- Brush mushroom caps with olive oil.
- Toss basil and tomatoes together, then season with pepper and salt and drizzle with olive oil. Allow to sit for a few minutes to let flavors merry.
- Place mushroom caps on the tray. Top with basil mixture and then mozzarella cheese.
- Bake just till cheese melted and caps are cooked.

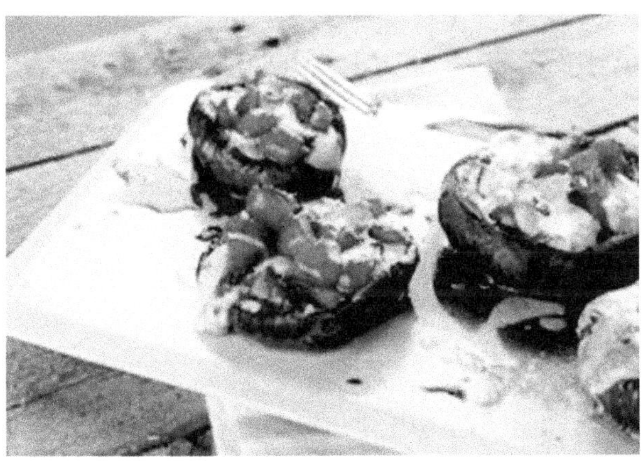

Mediterranean Meal Prep Chicken Bowls

What's in it:
- 1 ½ pounds thinly sliced grilled chicken
- 1 C. diced yellow and red bell peppers
- 20 kalamata olives
- 1 ¼ C. roasted chickpeas
- 5 ounces crumbled feta cheese
- ½ diced cucumber
- 20-25 haled grape tomatoes
- 5 handfuls spinach

Tahini Dressing:
- Pepper and salt
- 5 tbsp. water
- 3 tbsp. olive oil
- 4 tsp. lemon juice
- 1 minced garlic clove
- 5 tbsp. tahini

Roasted Chickpeas:
- Pepper and salt
- 2 tbsp. olive oil
- 15 ounce can drained/rinsed/dried chickpeas

How it's made:
- To make roasted chickpeas, ensure oven is preheated to 350 degrees.
- Toss peas with pepper, salt, and olive oil. Lay out in an even layer on a sheet and roast 20-30 minutes. Set to the side.
- Mix all of the dressing components together.
- To create bowls, put a handful of spinach into 5 containers.

- Top each container of spinach with 5 ounces chicken, 4 olives, ¼ C. roasted chickpeas, 1-ounce feta cheese, cucumber, and 4-5 tomatoes, and bell peppers.
- Add dressing over ingredients or pour into a dressing container.
- Chill bowls till ready to eat.

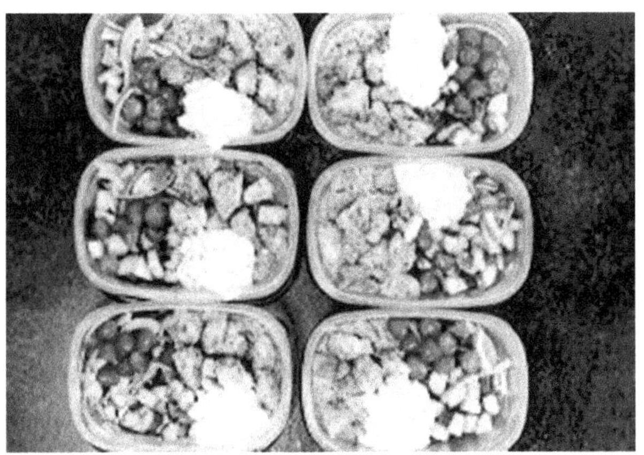

Mediterranean Cobb Salad

What's in it:

- 2 tbsp. basil
- ½ C. olives
- ¾ crumbled feta cheese
- ¾ diced cucumbers
- 1 C. marinated roasted red peppers
- 2 C. artichoke hearts
- 1-2 sliced hard-boiled eggs
- 4 C. romaine lettuce

Vinaigrette:

- ½ tsp. pepper
- ½ tsp. salt
- ½ tsp. drill
- ½ tsp. basil
- ½ tsp. oregano
- 1 tbsp. honey
- 1-2 tbsp. red wine vinegar
- 3-4 tbsp. olive oil

How it's made:

- Place romaine onto a platter and toss with remaining salad components till well combined.
- Add all vinaigrette ingredients to a bowl and mix vigorously. Drizzle over salad.

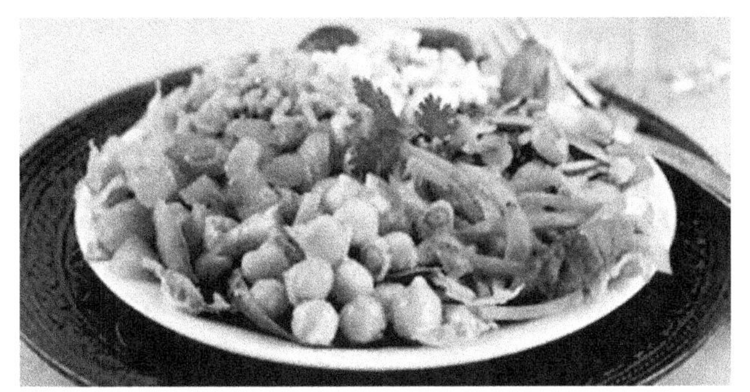

Avocado Veggie Quesadillas

What's in it:

- 1 C. shredded cheddar or mozzarella cheese
- 1 lime, sliced in half
- ¼ C. minced cilantro
- 2 avocados
- 1 tbsp. taco seasoning
- ½ C. drained black beans
- ½ sliced bell pepper
- ½ sliced onion

How it's made:

- Sauté bell pepper and onion together 2-3 minutes in a pan with 1 tbsp. heated oil till tenderized. Pour black beans into the pan and sprinkle everything with taco seasoning. Cook 60 seconds. Pour into a bowl and set to the side.
- Clean out the pan and heat up oil.
- Peel avocados and slice in half. Remove seed. Mash avocado with a fork. Season with pepper and salt and mix in lime juice and cilantro.
- Spread avocado mixture onto tortillas. Then spoon bean mixture on top along with ¼ cup of cheese.
- Fold tortilla. Cook 2-3 minutes on each side until crisp.
- Serve with sour cream and devour!

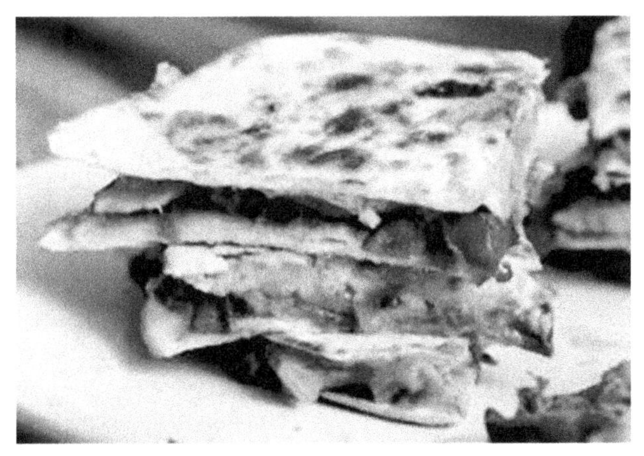

Grilled Chicken Greek Salad

What's in it:

Chicken:
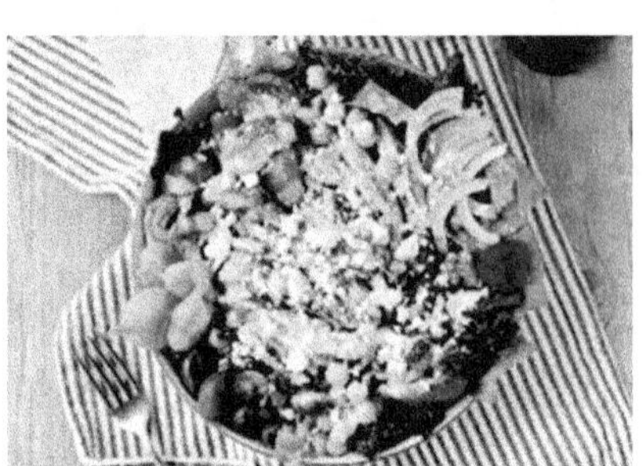
- Pepper and salt
- Mint
- Lemon rub
- Oregano
- Minced garlic
- 2 thin boneless chicken breasts

Salad:
- 1 C. crumbled feta cheese
- 1 C. kalamata olives
- 2 C. chopped tomatoes
- 2 sliced cucumbers
- ¼ sliced red onion
- Head romaine lettuce

Dressing:
- Pinch of pepper and salt
- ½ tsp. Greek herbs
- Juice of 1 ½ - 2 lemons
- ¼ C. extra virgin olive oil

How it's made:
- Ensure oven is preheated to 350 degrees.
- Preheat a grill. Brush chicken breasts with olive oil and sprinkle with chicken seasonings. Rub onto meat well.
- Grill chicken 2-3 minutes per side. Place chicken on sheet and bake 10-12 minutes.
- Pour lettuce into a salad bowl.

- Toss cheese, olives, tomatoes, cucumbers, and onions together.
  Whisk dressing components together till combined.
  Toss with veggies and cheese mixture.
- Add cheese mixture to romaine lettuce and toss gently. Top with grilled chicken. Drizzle with a bit more dressing when serving. Enjoy!

Turkey Taco Lettuce Wraps

What's in it:

- ½ C. shredded cheddar cheese
- 1 dollop sour cream
- 7-8 lettuce leaves
- 4-ounce tomato sauce
- ¾ C. water
- ½ minced onion
- 2 minced bell peppers
- ½ tsp. oregano
- 1 tsp. cumin
- 1 tsp. garlic powder
- 1 tsp. chili powder
- 1 tsp. salt
- 1 tsp. paprika
- 1 package ground turkey

How it's made:

- Heat oil and add turkey to pan. Break apart as it cooks, cooking till no longer pink. Pour in seasonings, combining well.
- Mix in tomato sauce, water, bell peppers, and onions. Let simmer 20 minutes.
- As turkey cooks, wash and dry lettuce.
- Place lettuce onto serving plates. Spoon turkey mixture into center of a lettuce leaf.
- Garnish with cheese and sour cream.

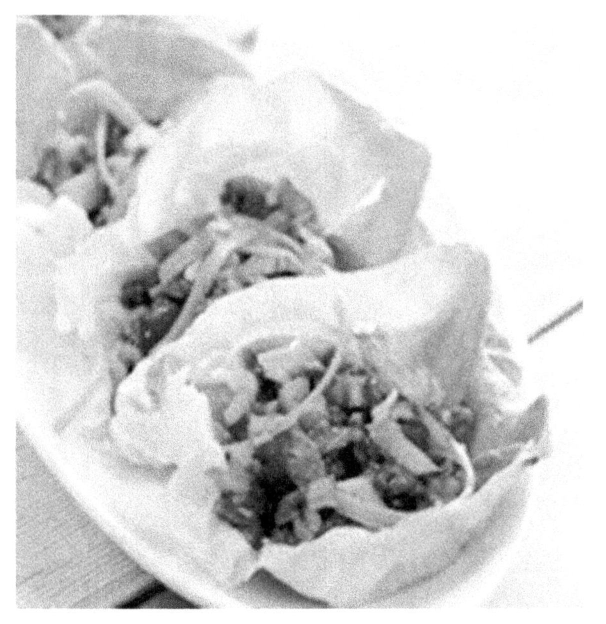

Mediterranean Flatbread

What's in it:
- Pepper
- ¼ C. arugula
- Sliced red onion
- 5 diced peperoncini peppers
- 1 tsp. olive oil
- ½ package halved grape tomatoes
- 1 Arugula Basil Pesto recipe
- 16 ounces pre-made pizza dough

Arugula Basil Pesto:
- Pepper and salt
- ¼ - ½ C. olive oil
- 1/3 C. whole unsalted cashews
- 1 garlic clove
- 1 C. basil
- 1 C. arugula

How it's made:
- To make pesto, place cashews, garlic, basil, and arugula into a food processor. Pulse till roughly chopped. Scrape sides.
- Drizzle olive oil into the processor, pulsing till you reach the consistency you like.
- Season with pepper and salt.
- Ensure oven is preheated to 420 degrees.
- Sprinkle flour onto a piece of parchment paper. Put pizza dough on parchment. Let dough sit 30 minutes to warm to room temperature.
- With foil, line a tray. Place tomatoes onto tray and brush with olive oil and sprinkle with oregano. Bake 8 minutes.

- Stretch out the dough. Place in oven on parchment paper 12 minutes.
- Take out the dough and spread pesto on top, along with red onion, pepperoncini peppers, and tomatoes.
- Pop back into the oven and bake 5 minutes.
- Top with pepper and arugula. Slice and devour!

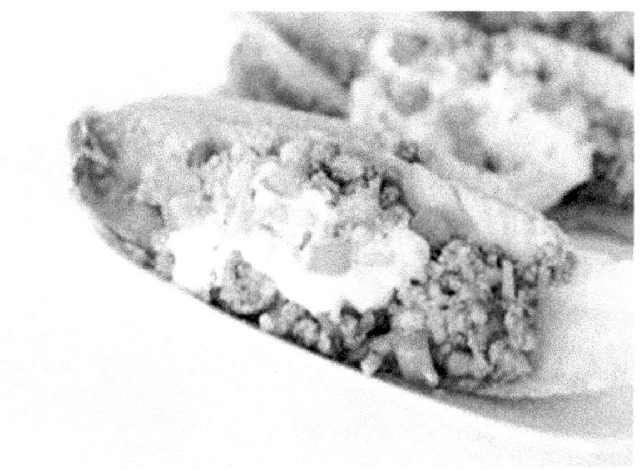

Grilled Lemon Herb Mediterranean Chicken Salad

What's in it:

Dressing and Marinade Mixture:
- Pepper
- 1 tsp. salt
- 1 tsp. oregano
- 2 tsp. minced garlic
- 2 tsp. basil
- 2 tbsp. chopped parsley
- 2 tbsp. red wine vinegar
- 2 tbsp. water
- Juice of 1 lemon
- 2 tbsp. olive oil
- 4 skinless, boneless chicken breasts

Salad:
- 1/3 C. kalamata olives
- 1 sliced avocado
- 1 sliced red onion
- 2 diced Roma tomatoes
- 1 diced cucumber
- 4 C. romaine lettuce
- Lemon wedges

How it's made:
- Combine all of dressing/marinade components together. Pour half of mixture into a dish and reserve rest. Add chicken to dish and marinade 2 hours.
- Toss all salad components in a bowl.
- Warm up oil and grill chicken until browned on all sides.

- Let chicken rest a few minutes before slicing.
- Arrange chicken over salad and drizzle with remaining dressing. Garnish with lemon wedges.

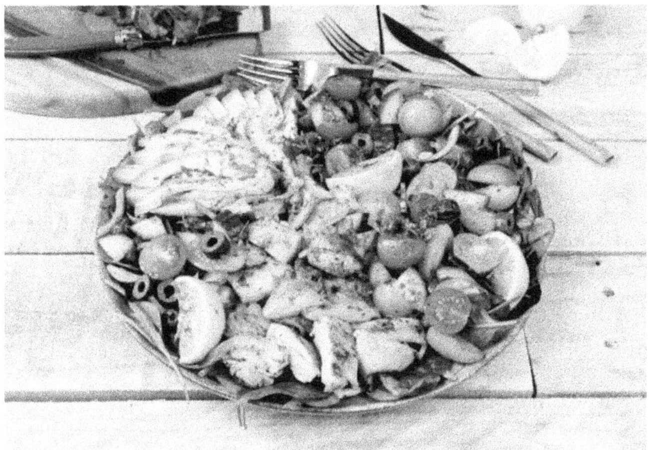

Mediterranean Chopped Salad Pitas

What's in it:

- 2 tbsp. dill
- ¾ C. crumbled feta
- ¾ C. chopped kalamata olives
- ½ diced red onion
- 1 diced cucumber
- 1 diced tomato
- 15 ounce can chickpeas (drained/rinsed)
- 1 head chopped romaine lettuce
- Pita bread

Dressing:

- ¼ tsp. pepper
- ½ tsp. salt
- ½ tsp. Italian seasoning
- 2 tbsp. red wine vinegar
- ¼ C. olive oil

How it's made:

- Whisk all dressing components together.
- Add salad components to a bowl and toss well. Drizzle dressing and toss once more before adding to pita bread. Yum!

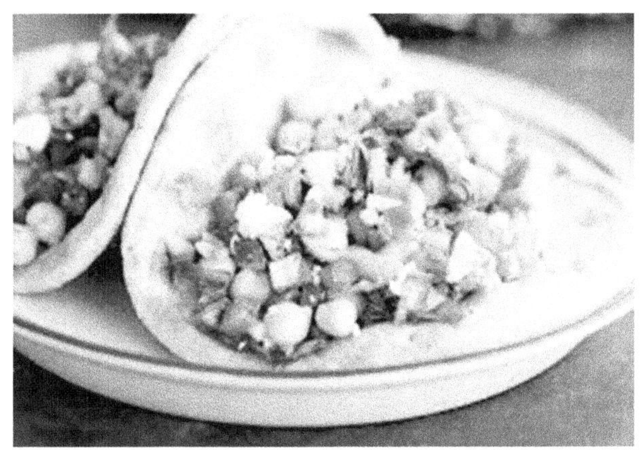

Snack and Appetizer Recipes

Easy Mediterranean Layer Dip

What's in it:

- ¼ C. crumbled feta cheese
- ¼ C. chopped sun-dried tomatoes
- ¼ C. sliced black olives
- 1 chopped cucumber
- ½ C. pesto
- 1 C. hummus

How it's made:

- Spread hummus in a single layer onto a serving platter.
- Next, pour pesto over hummus, smoothing out evenly.
- Sprinkle feta cheese, tomatoes, olive, and cucumber over pesto.
- Serve dip with crackers, raw vegetables, and pita chips!

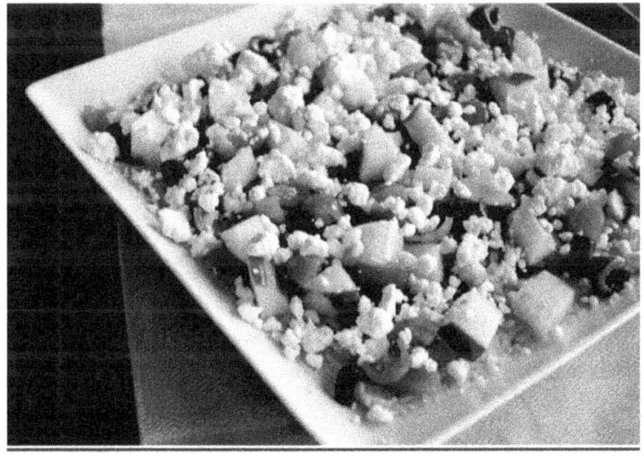

Stuffed Mushrooms

What's in it:

- 1 quartered lemon
- 5 ounces feta cheese
- ½ tsp. paprika
- ½ tsp. onion powder
- ½ tsp. garlic powder
- ½ tsp. salt
- ½ tsp. pepper
- ½ tsp. Italian seasoning
- 5 tbsp. olive oil
- 5 portobello mushrooms caps
- 2/3 C. chopped mixed jarred antipasto mix

How it's made:

- Take out the middle of mushrooms caps and toss with spices and olive oil.
- Warm up pan and grill mushrooms with lemons for 10 minutes.
- Mix antipasto and feta cheese together.
- Stuff mushrooms caps with feta cheese mixture and grill 2-3 more minutes.
- Garnish with parsley and a nice squeeze from the charred lemons.

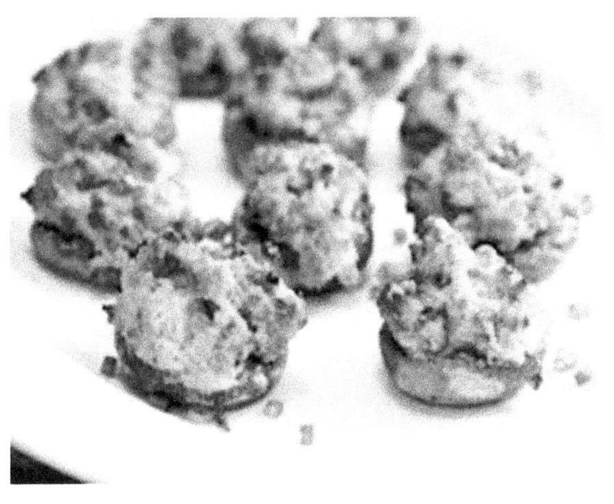

Hummus Quesadillas

What's in it:

- ¼ C. hummus
- 1 C. baby spinach leaves
- ¼ C. diced roasted red peppers
- 1 diced garlic cloves
- ¼ tsp. olive oil
- Whole wheat tortilla
- Pepper and salt

How it's made:

- Warm up oil and sauté red peppers and garlic together 2-3 minutes, sprinkling with pepper and salt.
- Place spinach and pan and cook 60 seconds.
- Wipe out pan and place tortilla into it. Spread hummus onto half of tortilla. Top with red pepper mixture. Fold in half, cooking till browned on both sides.
- Slice and eat!

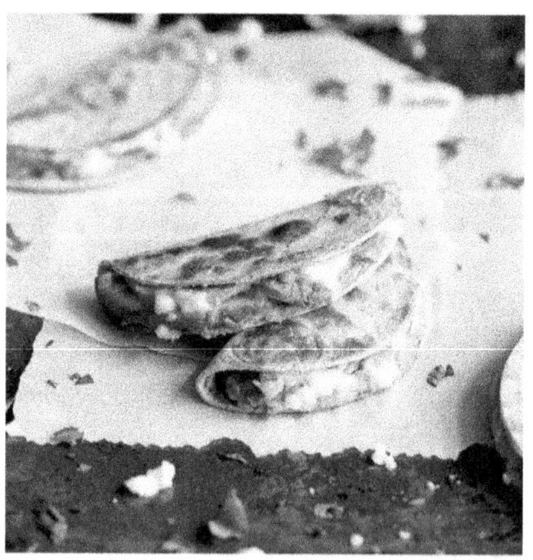

Marinated Olives with Feta

What's in it:

- Pepper
- Pinch of crushed red pepper
- 1 tsp. rosemary
- 2 sliced garlic cloves
- Juice and zest of 1 lemon
- 2 tbsp. extra virgin olive oil
- ½ C. diced feta cheese
- 1 C. sliced Greek olives

How it's made:

- Mix all recipe components together in a bowl, tossing well to combine.
- Serve with crackers!

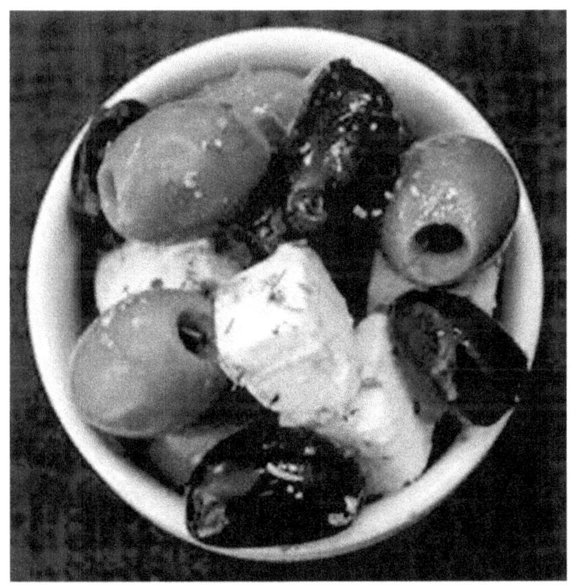

Tomato and Basil Finger Sandwiches

What's in it:

- 1/8 tsp. pepper
- 1/8 tsp. salt
- 4 tsp. basil
- 4 thick slices of tomato
- 8 tsp. reduced-fat mayo
- 4 slices whole wheat bread

How it's made:

- Cut bread into rounds that are just a bit bigger than slices of tomato.
- Spread slices of bread with 2 tsp. mayo. Top with pepper, salt, basil, and tomatoes.

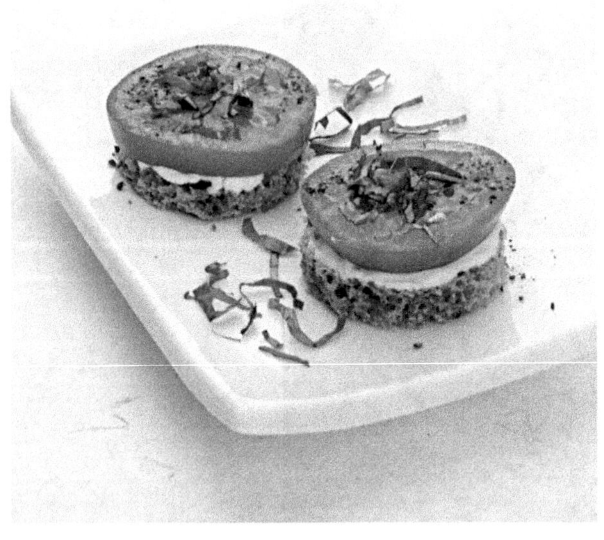

Herbed Olives

What's in it:

- 2 tsp. extra virgin olive oil
- 3 C. olives of choice
- Pepper
- 1 crushed garlic clove
- 1/8 tsp. basil
- 1/8 tsp. oregano

How it's made:

- Toss olives with pepper, garlic, basil, and oregano till well combined.

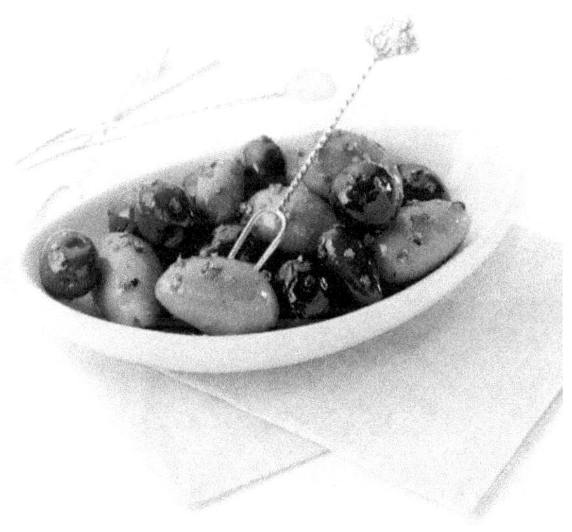

Date Wraps

What's in it:

- Pepper
- 16 whole pitted dates
- 16 thin slices Prosciutto

How it's made:

- Wrap dates with a slice of Prosciutto.
- Season with pepper. Enjoy!

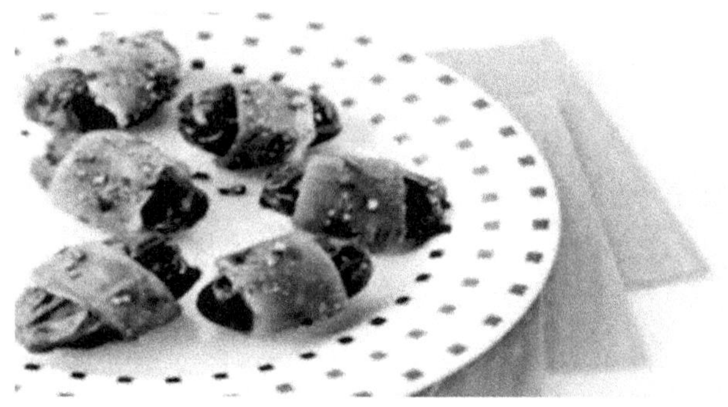

Blueberries with Lemon Cream

What's in it:

- 2 C. fresh blueberries
- 2 tsp. grated lemon zest
- 1 tsp. honey
- ¾ C. low-fat vanilla yogurt
- 4 ounces cream cheese (preferably reduced-fat)

How it's made:

- Break up cream cheese with a fork.
  Drain liquid from yogurt and combine with honey and
  cream cheese. Beat with electric mixer until creamy.
  Mix in lemon zest.
- Into dishes, layer lemon cream, and blueberries.
- A sweet treat!

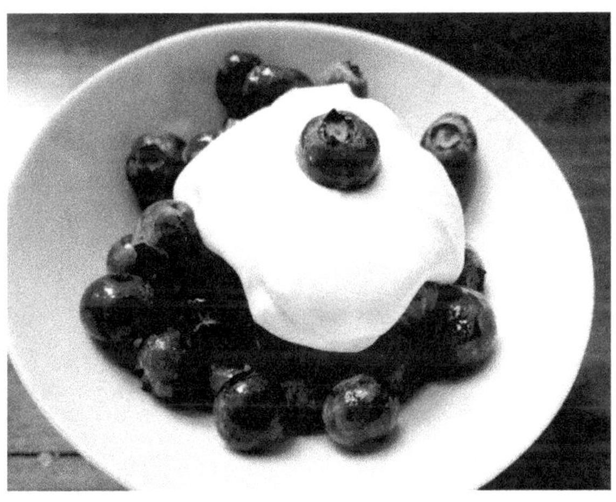

Tomato and Basil Skewers

What's in it:

- Pepper and salt
- Extra virgin olive oil
- 16 cherry tomatoes
- 16 basil leaves
- 16 small mozzarella balls

How it's made:

- Thread tomatoes, basil, and mozzarella balls onto skewers.
- Drizzle with olive oil and season with pepper and salt.

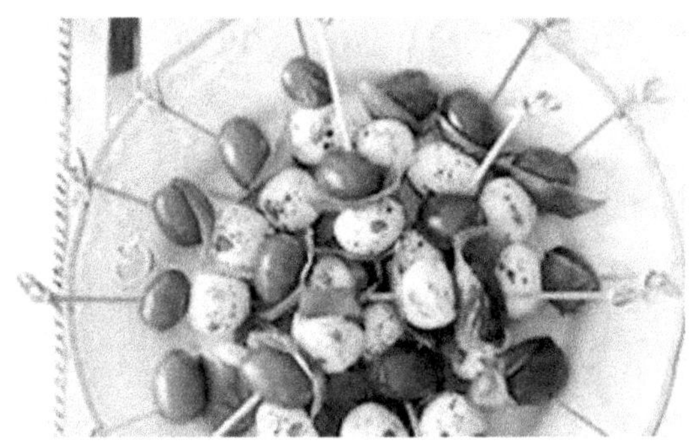

Cherries with Ricotta and Toasted Almonds

What's in it:

- 1 tbsp. toasted slivered almonds
- 2 tbsp. ricotta cheese
- ¾ C. frozen pitted cherries

How it's made:

- Warm cherries in microwave 1-2 minutes.
- Top warmed up cherries with almonds and ricotta cheese. Enjoy!

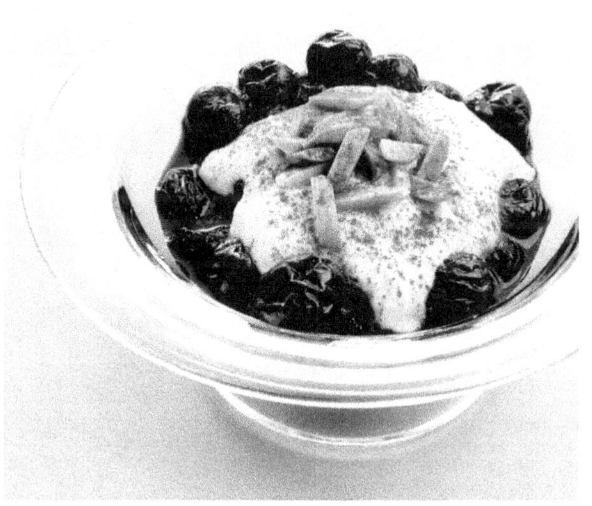

Side Recipes

Tzatziki Cucumber Salad

What's in it:

- 3 cucumbers
- Juice of ½ a lemon
- Pepper
- ½ tsp. salt
- 2 tsp. olive oil
- 1-2 tbsp. chopped dill
- 1 minced garlic clove
- ¼ C. plain Greek yogurt

How it's made:

- Combine all recipe components together, except cucumber. Cover with plastic wrap and chill 1 hour.
- Wash cucumbers and cut into slices.
- Pour cucumber slices into bowl yogurt dressing and toss well. Serve cold!

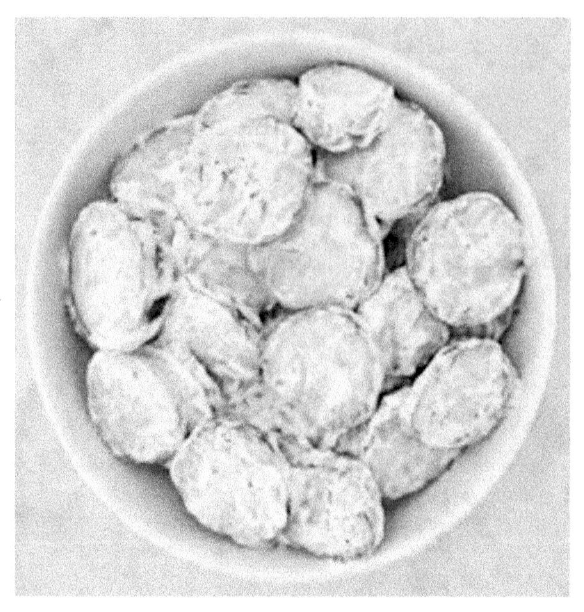

Mediterranean Brussels Sprouts

What's in it:

- 1 C. tri-colored rotini pasta
- ¼ C. crumbled feta cheese
- Cracked peppercorns
- Pepper and salt
- ¼ C. extra virgin olive oil
- 1 bay leaf
- 2 tsp. pine nuts
- ½ C. kalamata olives
- 5 sun-dried tomato pieces
- 2 C. Brussels sprouts

How it's made:

- Ensure oven is preheated to 350 degrees.
- Clean and dry Brussels sprouts. Cut up tomatoes and cook rotini pasta.
- Warm up olive oil. Place sprouts into the pan, sprinkle with salt and cook 7-8 minutes. Then place in oven and bake 10 minutes.
- As sprouts bake, heat up a pan with remaining oil. Add tomatoes and olives, cooking 5 minutes.
- Take sprouts from oven and pour into olive mixture.
- Place pan into the oven and bake an additional 10 minutes.
  Sprinkle with feta cheese
- Roast pine nuts and top sprouts with them.

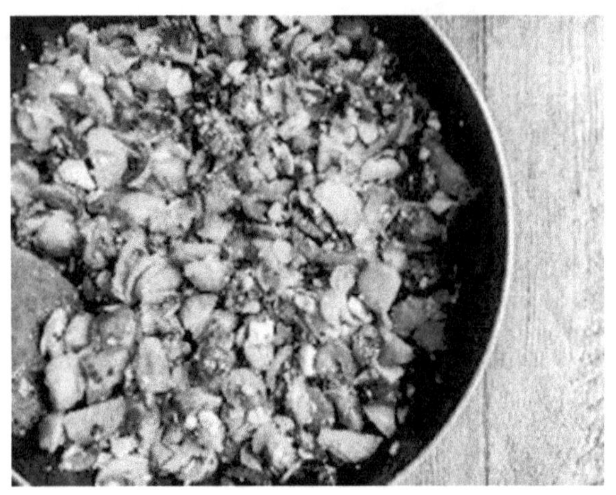

Parmesan Sun-Dried Tomato and Basil Rice

What's in it:

- ½ C. shredded parmesan cheese
- 10 chopped basil leaves
- ½ C. drained/chopped sun-dried tomatoes
- ¼ tsp. salt
- 1 C. uncooked Jasmine rice
- 2 C. chicken broth

How it's made:

- Add salt, uncooked rice, and chicken broth into a pan. Warm to boiling. Turn down heat and let simmer 15-20 minutes till rice is cooked.
- Take the pan off the heat and add tomatoes, drained oil, and basil along with parmesan cheese.
- Combine everything till incorporated.
- Season with salt and olive oil.
- Serve garnished with basil.

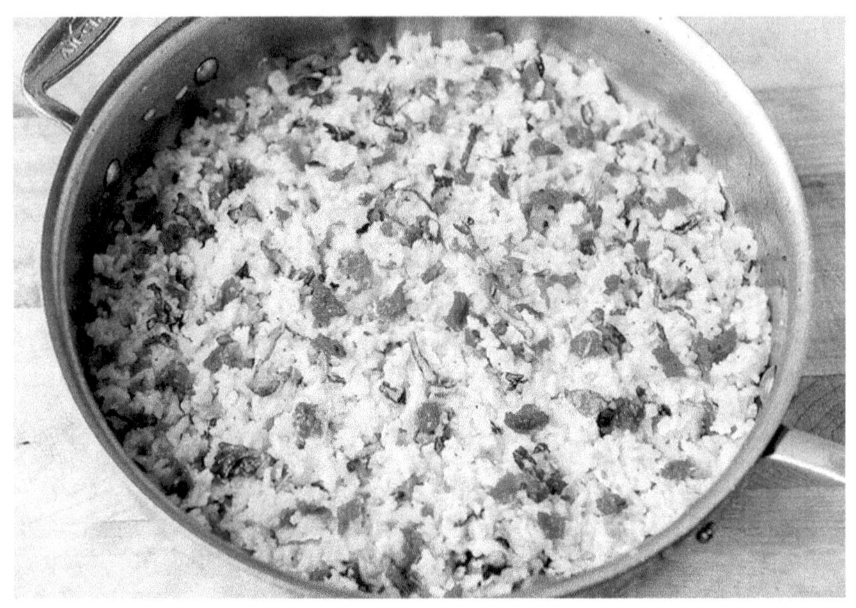

Mediterranean Rice Pilaf

What's in it:

- 1 chopped tomato
- ½ tsp. paprika
- 1 C. chickpeas
- 1 tsp. tomato paste
- 1 package basmati rice
- 1 minced garlic
- 1 chopped onion
- ½ chopped red bell pepper
- ½ chopped yellow bell pepper
- ½ chopped green bell pepper
- 1 tbsp. olive oil

How it's made:

- Sauté garlic, onions, and peppers with olive oil until tender. Then mix in chickpeas, tomato paste, and rice.
- Combine well and add salt and paprika.
- Top with tomatoes and serve topped with parsley.

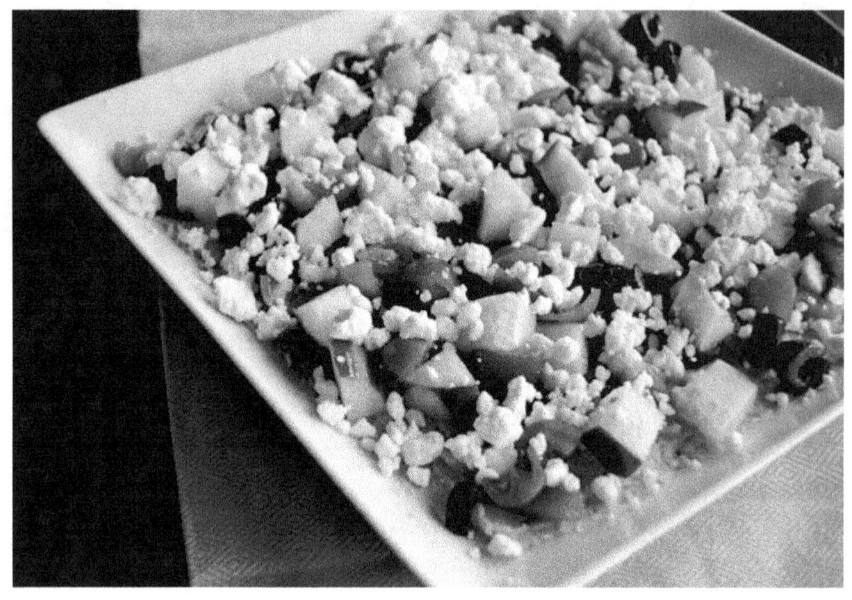

Turmeric Roasted Carrots

What's in it:

- Juice of ½ a lime
- Pepper and salt
- 3 minced garlic cloves
- ½ tsp. coriander
- 1 tsp. cinnamon
- 1 tsp. turmeric
- Extra virgin olive oil
- 3 pounds peeled whole carrots

How it's made:

- Ensure oven is preheated to 400 degrees.
- Place carrots in a single layer on a tray. Toss with minced garlic, pepper, salt, spices, and olive oil.
- Bake 40-45 minutes till carrots are tender.
- Serve garnished with parsley and dill.

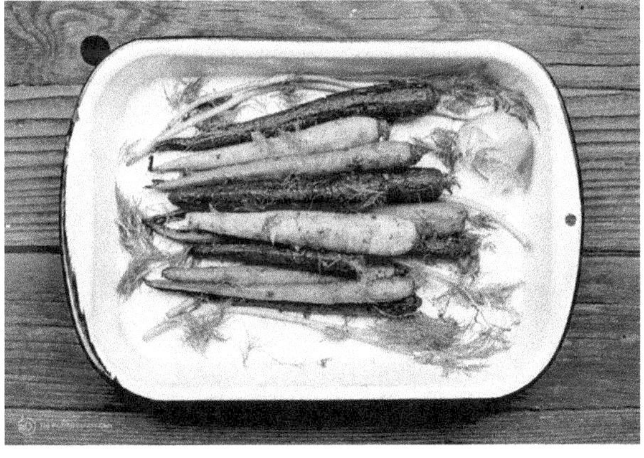

Roasted Mediterranean Potatoes

What's in it:

- 1 tbsp. chopped Italian parsley
- 1/8 C. crumbled feta cheese
- ¼ C. caramelized onions
- Pinch of salt
- 1 tsp. chopped thyme
- 1 tbsp. chopped rosemary
- 2 minced cloves garlic
- 1 tbsp. olive oil
- 1 pound red or baby potatoes (sliced into bite-sized pieces)

How it's made:

- Ensure oven is preheated to 400 degrees.
- Toss potatoes with olive oil, thyme, rosemary, and garlic.
- Spread potato mixture on a tray and season with salt. Top with onions.
- Bake 20-25 minutes until tender.
- Allow to cool 5 minutes before serving with feta cheese and parsley.

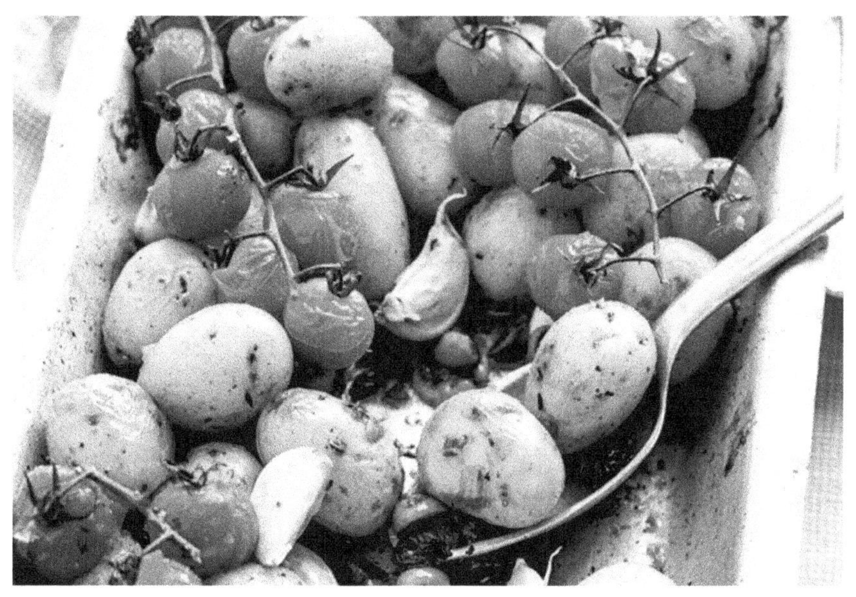

Roasted Eggplant

What's in it:

- Toasted pine nuts
- ½ C. pomegranate seeds
- ½ C. chopped parsley
- ½ tbsp. za'atar spice
- Olive oil
- Salt
- 1 eggplant

How it's made:

- Slice eggplant into ¾ inch rounds. Place slices onto tray and season with salt. Let sit half an hour to sweat out the bitterness.
- Ensure oven is preheated to 400 degrees.
- Dry eggplant with paper towels and lightly brush with olive oil.
- Bake 35-40 minutes until golden.
- Take out of the oven and sprinkle with za'atar seasoning.
- Garnish with pine nuts, pomegranate seeds, and parsley.

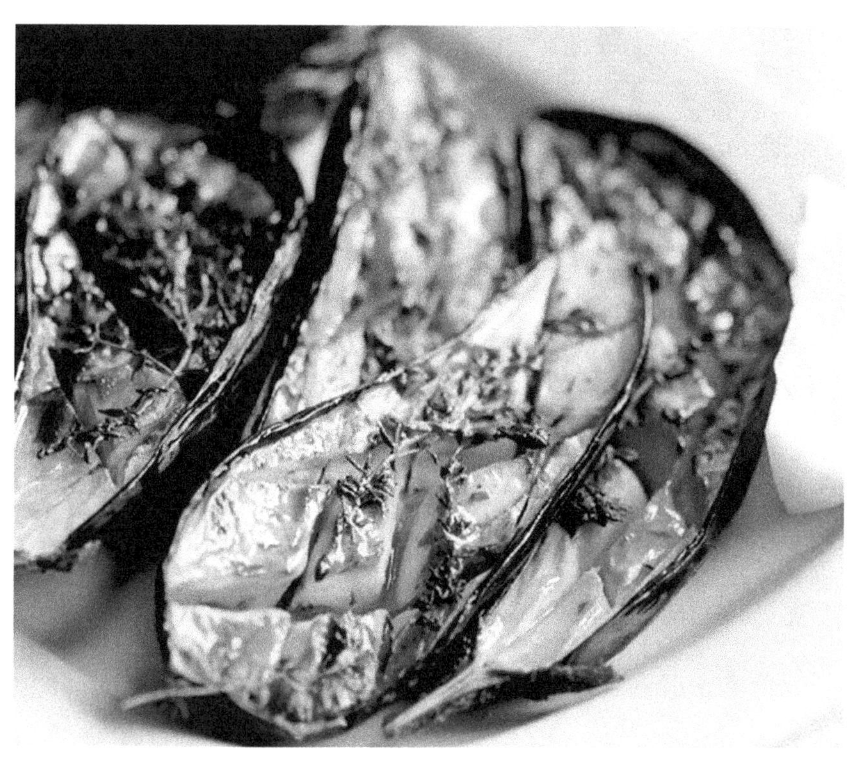

Italian Oven Roasted Veggies

What's in it:

- Pepper and salt
- 1 tsp. thyme
- ½ tbsp. oregano
- Olive oil
- 10-12 peeled garlic cloves
- 2 zucchini
- 12 ounces Campari tomatoes
- 12 ounces baby potatoes
- 8 ounces bella mushrooms
- Grated parmesan cheese
- Crushed red pepper flakes

How it's made:

- Clean and trim mushrooms. Scrub and half potatoes. Slice zucchini into 1-inch pieces.
- Ensure oven is preheated 425 degrees.
- Pour garlic, veggies, and mushrooms into a bowl and toss. Add pepper, salt, thyme, oregano, drizzling with olive oil and tossing well.
- Spread evenly onto the tray.
- Roast 20-25 minutes until tender.
- Serve with parmesan cheese and red pepper flakes.

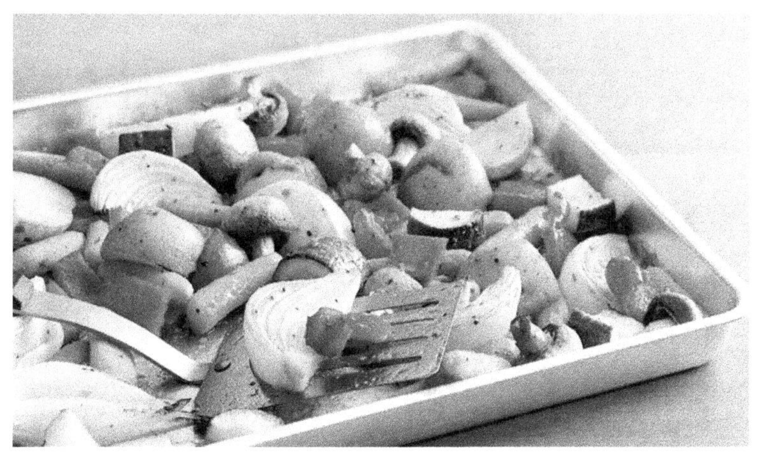

Mediterranean Spaghetti Squash

What's in it:

- Pepper and salt
- 3 tbsp. chopped basil
- ½ C. sliced black olives
- ¾ C. crumbled feta cheese
- 2 ½ C. halved grape tomatoes
- 1 minced garlic clove
- 1 chopped onion
- 2 tbsp. vegetable oil
- 3-4 pounds spaghetti squash

How it's made:

- Cut squash in half lengthwise and remove seeds.
- Ensure oven is preheated to 350 degrees. Grease a tray lightly.
- Put squash, cut side down, onto the tray. Bake 35-45 minutes until tender.
- Sauté onion in heated oil. Add garlic and sauté 30 seconds. Then mix in tomatoes, heating 60 seconds.
- Shred squash with forks, creating strands.
- Toss sautéed veggies with basil, olives, and feta cheese. Season with pepper and salt and serve warm.

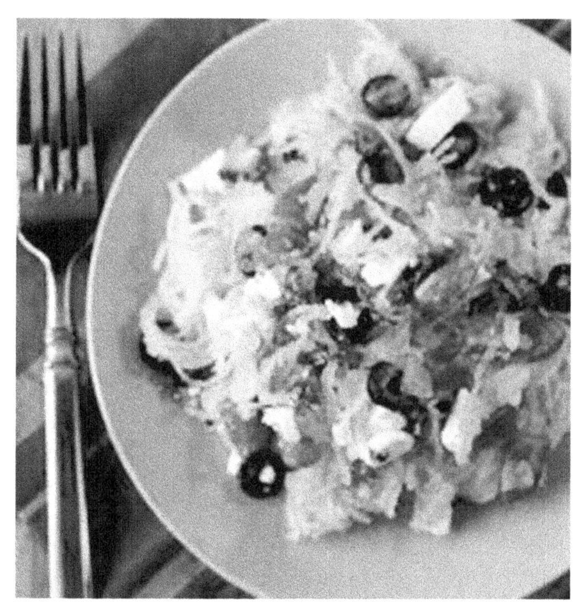

Garlic Cauliflower

What's in it:

- 2 tbsp. oil
- 1 tbsp. paprika
- Salt
- 1 tbsp. onion powder
- 1 tbsp. garlic powder
- 1 potato
- 1 small head cauliflower

How it's made:

- Ensure oven is preheated to 400 degrees.
- Cut potato and break up cauliflower. Slice into florets. Toss with salt, spices, and oil. Place onto a tray.
- Bake 25 minutes till cauliflower is crisp.
- Pour into a bowl and garnish with cilantro and a squeeze of lime.

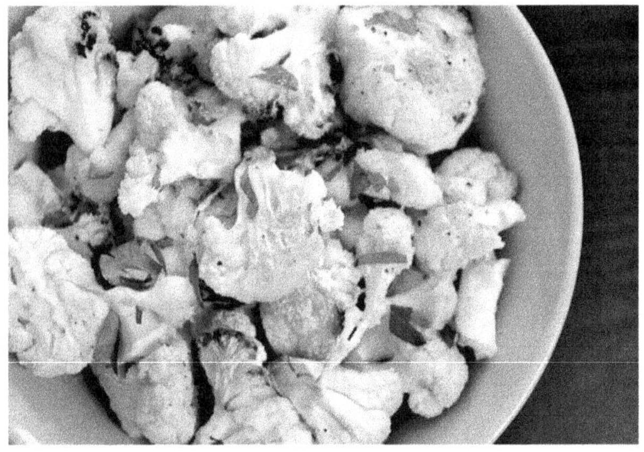

Soup and Stew Recipes

Mediterranean Kale, Cannellini, and Farro Stew

What's in it:

- Crumbled feta cheese
- 1 tbsp. lime juice
- 15 ounce can cannellini beans (drained and rinsed)
- 4 C. kale
- ½ C. parsley sprigs
- Salt
- 1 bay lea
- 1 tsp. oregano
- 1 C. rinsed farro
- 14.5 ounce can diced tomatoes
- 5 C. low-sodium vegetable broth
- 1 C. chopped celery
- 1 C. chopped yellow onion
- 1 C. diced carrots
- 2 tbsp. olive oil

How it's made:

- Warm oil in a pan and sauté celery, onions, and carrots 3 minutes. Add garlic, then sauté 30 seconds. Pour in vegetable broth and stir in bay leaf, oregano, farro, and tomatoes. Season with salt.
- Lay parsley into a mound on top of soup and heat to boiling.
  Turn down heat and simmer covered 20 minutes. Remove parsley and stir in kale. Cook 10-15 minutes, then add cannellini beans. Cook until kale and farro are tenderized.
- Take out the bay leaf and mix in lemon juice.

- Serve warm with feta cheese.

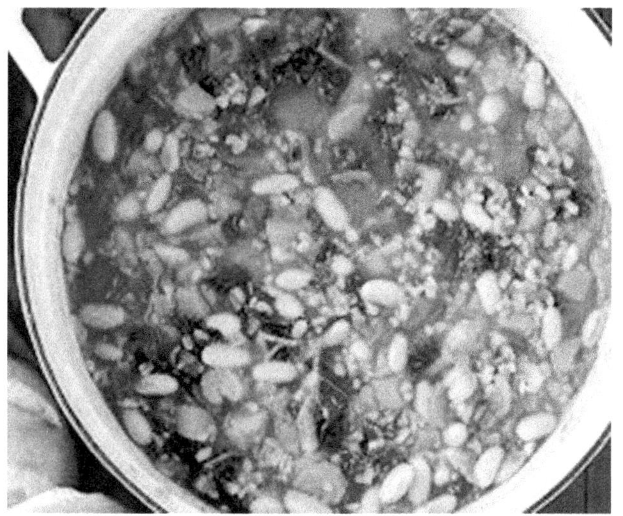

Shrimp Orzo Soup

What's in it:
- Juice of 1 lemon
- 1 C. chopped dill
- 1 C. chopped parsley
- 6 ounces baby spinach
- 1 C. orzo pasta
- 3 diced tomatoes
- 7 C. vegetable broth
- 1 tbsp. oregano
- 3 tbsp. tomato paste
- 6 peeled/minced garlic cloves
- 1 chopped yellow onion
- 1 chopped red bell pepper
- 1 chopped green bell pepper
- 1 ½ pounds shrimp
- Olive oil
- Pepper and salt
- 8 ounces scallops
- Crushed red pepper flakes

How it's made:
- Season scallops with pepper and salt.
- Warm up oil and add scallops. Sear 1-2 minutes until golden. Sprinkle with oregano. Add shrimp, searing till pink, Add ½ of oregano.
- In a pot, warm oil and add salt, remaining oregano, tomato paste, garlic, onions, and peppers. Cook 5 minutes.
- Pour in vegetable broth and bring mixture to boiling. Add tomatoes and cook 3-5 minutes.
- Pour in pasta, turn down heat and cook 8 minutes, until tender.

- Mix in lemon juice, dill, parsley, and baby spinach.
- Add shrimp and scallops. Cook just till warmed through. Season with pepper, salt, and red pepper flakes to achieve desired taste.
- Serve with crusty bread and enjoy!

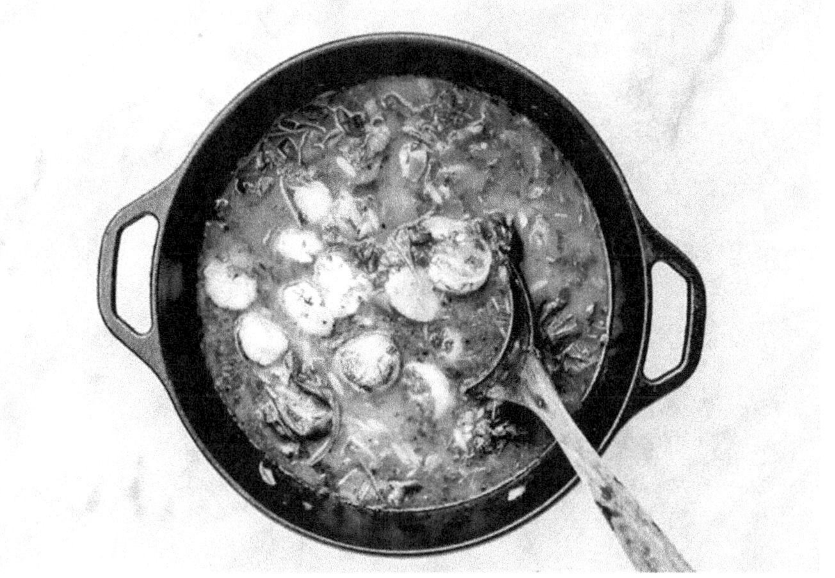

Chicken Orzo Soup

What's in it:

- 1 tbsp. lemon juice
- 1 tsp. lemon peel
- 1 C. uncooked whole wheat orzo pasta
- 1 bay leaf
- 1 tsp. minced rosemary
- 32 ounces reduced-sodium chicken broth
- ¼ C. white wine
- ¼ tsp. pepper
- ½ tsp. oregano
- ½ tsp. salt
- 1 chopped onion
- 2 chopped carrots
- 2 chopped celery ribs
- ¾ pound boneless skinless chicken breasts, cut into cubes
- 2 tbsp. olive oil

How it's made:

- Warm up half of oil and add chicken, cooking 6-8 minutes till cooked. Take out of the pan.
- Heat remaining oil and add pepper, oregano, salt, and veggies, cooking 4-6 minutes until tender but slightly crisp. Pour in wine to loosen bits from pan. Mix in bay leaf, rosemary, and broth. Bring mixture to a boil.
- Pour in orzo, turn down heat and let simmer 15-18 minutes till orzo is tender and cooked.
- Place chicken back in the pan and then mix in lemon juice and peel. Trash bay leaf.
- Garnish soup with parsley when serving.

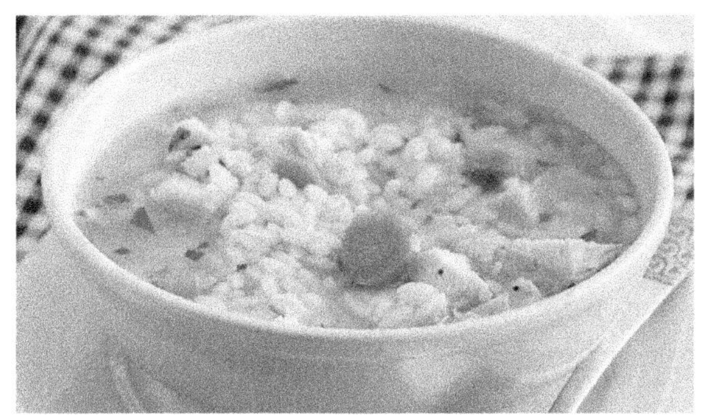

Spicy Spinach Lentil Soup

What's in it:

- 2 C. chopped parsley
- Juice of 1 lime
- 1 ½ C. rinsed brown lentils
- 12 ounces frozen spinach
- 3 C. water
- 6 C. low-sodium vegetable broth
- 1 tbsp. flour
- Pinch of sugar
- 2 tsp. mint flakes
- 1 ½ tsp. crushed red peppers
- 1 ½ tsp. sumac
- 1 ½ tsp. cumin
- 1 ½ tsp. coriander
- Pepper and salt
- 1 chopped garlic clove
- 1 chopped yellow onion
- Extra virgin olive oil

How it's made:

- Heat 2 tbsp olive oil and sauté onions until brown. Then add flour, sugar, mint, spices, and garlic, cooking 2 minutes.
- Pour in water and broth. Turn up the heat to make mixture boil and add lentils and spinach. Cook 5 minutes.
- Turn down heat, cover and cook 20 minutes till lentils become tender.
- Stir in parsley and lime juice. Let mixture sit covered 5 minutes.

- Serve hot with pita bread!

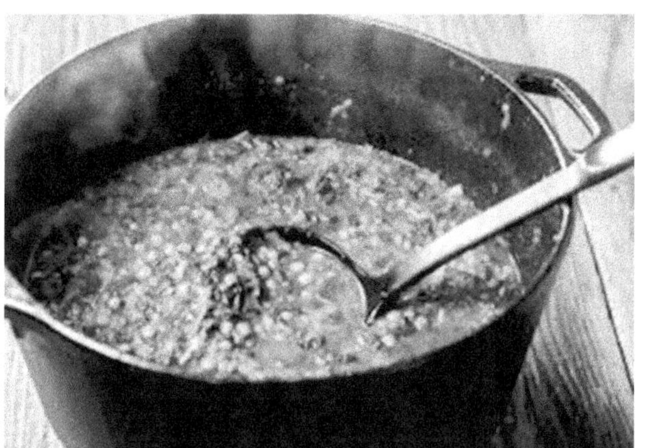

Creamy Tuscan Garlic Tortellini Soup

What's in it:

- 2 C. spinach
- 9 ounces tortellini
- 2 C. cooked/shredded chicken
- ¼ tsp. pepper
- 1 tbsp. Italian seasoning
- ¼ C. parmesan cheese
- 1 C. heavy cream
- 15 ounce can white beans (drained and rinsed)
- 28 ounce can diced tomatoes
- 4 C. chicken broth
- 3 minced cloves garlic
- 1 diced onion
- 2 tbsp. butter

How it's made:

- Warm butter and sauté garlic and onion until tender.
- Pour in pepper, salt, Italian seasoning, parmesan cheese, heavy cream, white beans, tomatoes, and chicken broth. Heat to simmering.
- Add spinach, tortellini, and chicken. Simmer 10 minutes for the mixture to thicken.

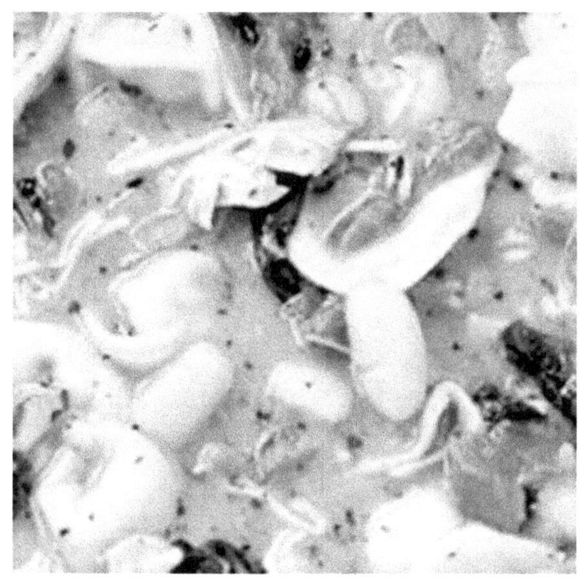

Vegetable Barley Soup

What's in it:
- Pepper and salt
- 1/3 C chopped Italian parsley
- 2/3 C. frozen peas
- 1 bay leaf
- ½ tsp. oregano
- 1 tsp. basil
- 2/3 C. frozen corn
- 1 C. pearl barley
- 1 ½ C. frozen cut green beans
- 14.5 ounce can diced tomatoes
- 15 ounce can drained and rinsed chickpeas
- 8 C. vegetable broth
- 2 minced garlic cloves
- 1 sliced celery stalk
- 2 sliced carrots
- 8 ounces sliced mushrooms
- 1 diced onion
- 1 tbsp. extra virgin olive oil

How it's made:
- Warm up oil and sauté celery, carrots, and onions together 5 minutes till softened, seasoning with pepper and salt.
- Turn up the heat and add mushrooms, cook till browned. Stir in garlic, cooking 30 seconds.
- Add bay leaf, oregano, basil, corn, barley, green beans, tomatoes, chickpeas, and broth. Bring the mixture up to boiling, then reduce heat to a simmer.
- Cook 30 minutes until tender.
- Stir in peas and trash bay leaf. Mix in parsley and season with pepper and salt.

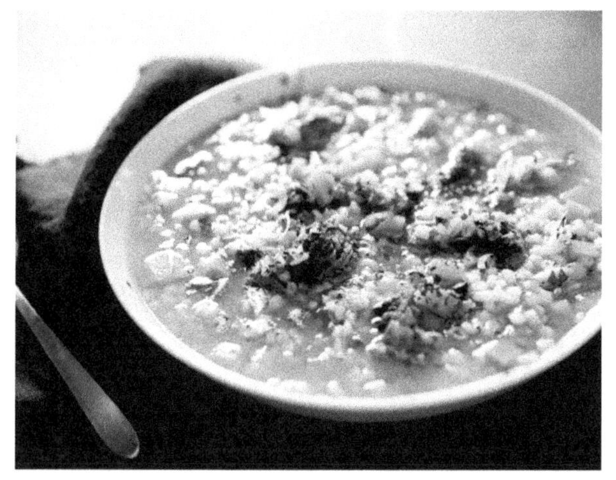

Pumpkin Soup

What's in it:

- Pinch of salt
- 2 tsp. pepper
- 8 ½ C. vegetable broth
- Half of cabbage head
- 2 potatoes
- 6 peeled/crushed garlic cloves
- 1 sliced leek
- 2 chopped carrots
- 1 de-seeded, peeled, and cut pumpkin
- 2 tbsp. extra virgin olive oil

How it's made:

- Heat up oil and sweat veggies for 10 minutes.
  Pour in stock and heat to boiling. Simmer 25 minutes
  till veggies are softened.
- With an immersion blender, blend mixture until
  smooth. Season with pepper and salt to achieve
  desired taste.
- Spoon into bowls and eat warm, or chill and consume
  cold.

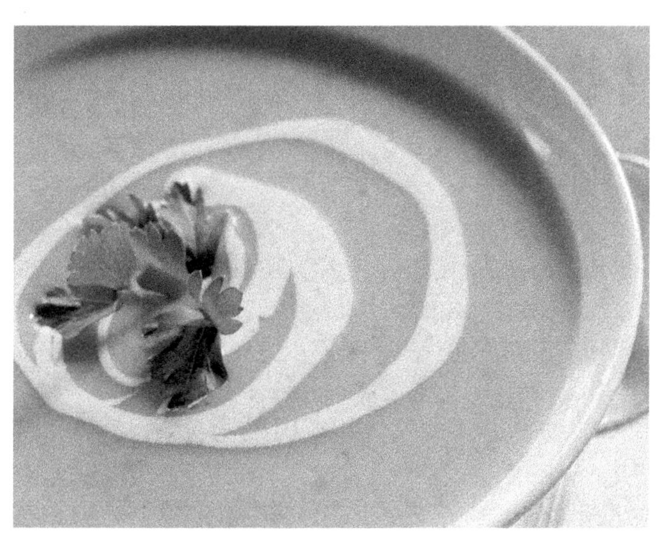

Greek Bean Soup

What's in it:

- ½ C. chopped parsley
- 1 zested and juiced lemon
- ¼ tsp. cayenne pepper
- ¼ tsp. sweet paprika
- ½ tsp. cumin
- 3 15-ounce cans cannellini beans (drained and rinsed)
- 4 ½ C. chicken broth
- 1 tsp. oregano
- 1 bay leaf
- 4 chopped celery ribs
- 2 minced garlic cloves
- ½ tsp. pepper
- ½ tsp. salt
- 1 chopped yellow onion
- Extra virgin olive oil

How it's made:

- Warm up olive oil. Add pepper, salt, and onion. Cook 4 minutes. Then add oregano, bay leaf, celery, and garlic. Cook another 5 minutes.
- Then pour in broth, along with cayenne pepper, paprika, cumin, and cannelloni beans.
- Turn up the heat and boil 3 minutes. Turn down heat and simmer 10 minutes.
- Spoon 2 cups of soup into a food processor. Blend and pour back into the pot. Simmer 5 minutes.
- Take off heat and stir in 1/3 cup olive oil, along with parsley, lemon juice, and lemon zest.
- Serve with crusty bread.

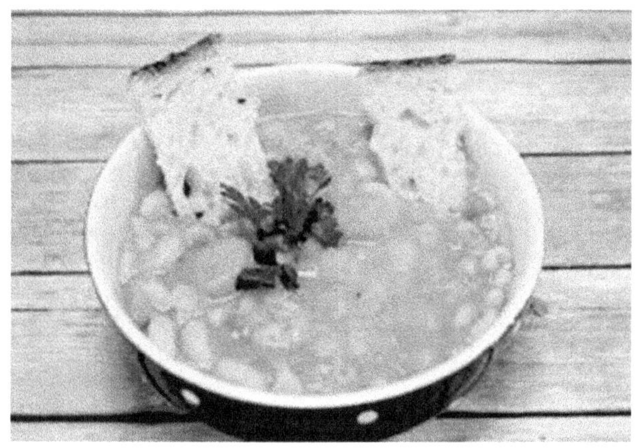

Moroccan Meatball Couscous Soup

What's in it:

Meatballs:
- 1 ½ pounds lamb or beef
- 2 tbsp. tomato paste
- Pepper and salt
- ¼ tsp. chili powder
- 1/8 tsp. nutmeg
- 1/8 tsp. cinnamon
- ¼ tsp. turmeric
- ½ tsp. thyme
- ½ tsp. curry powder
- 1 tsp. cumin
- 1 tsp. coriander

Soup:
- 3 ¾ C. water
- 4 C. chicken broth
- 8 minced cloves garlic
- 3 minced shallots
- 3 tbsp. + 2 tsp. olive oil
- 8 ounces pearl couscous

How it's made:
- Ensure oven is preheated to 375 degrees. With parchment paper, line a tray.
- Mix meatball spices, pepper, and salt together. Then add meat and tomato paste. Create meatballs and place onto the sheet. Bake 10-12 minutes.
- As meatballs cook, warm up oil and add couscous, toasting 1-2 minutes.

- Then add 1 ¾ cups water and salt. Turn down heat and simmer 8-10 minutes.
- In a Dutch oven, heat 3 tbsp. oil and add garlic and shallots, sauté for 1 minute.
- Pour in chicken broth and remaining water, bringing to a boil.
- Turn down heat and simmer 10 minutes.
- Spoon into serving bowls with mint.

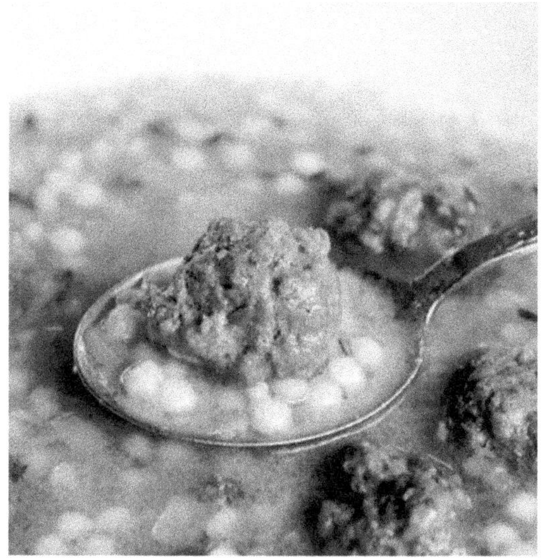

Roasted Butternut Squash Soup

What's in it:

- Pepper and salt
- 6 C. chicken broth
- 1 chopped onion
- 2 tbsp. unsalted butter
- 1 tbsp. olive oil
- 2-3 pounds peeled/seeded butternut squash

How it's made:

- Ensure oven is preheated to 400 degrees.
- Slice squash in half and remove seeds. Drizzle with olive oil.
- Lay squash down, face down onto a tray.
- Bake 40-50 minutes until tender. Allow to cool.
- Remove pulp and skin. Chop into chunks.
- Melt butter and sauté onion till translucent.
- Place squash with chicken broth. Pour into blender and blender until smooth.
- Season with pepper and salt.

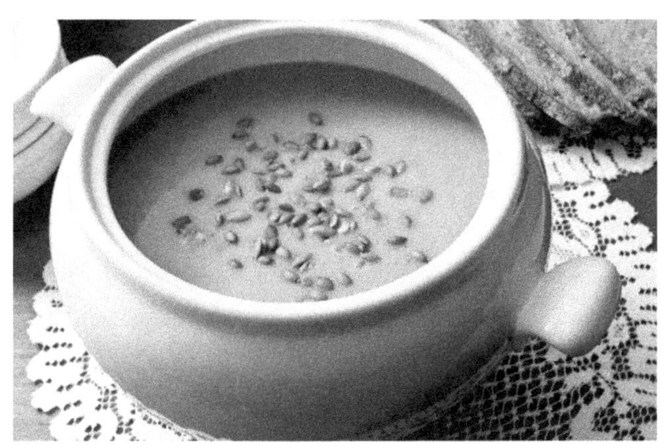

Dinner Recipes

One-Pan Lemon Herb Chicken and Potatoes

What's in it:

- 4 tbsp. kalamata olives
- 1 sliced zucchini
- 1 sliced red bell pepper
- 1 onion, cut into wedges
- 8 halved baby potatoes
- 2 tsp. salt
- 2 tsp. parsley
- 2 tsp. oregano
- 3 tsp. basil
- 4 crushed garlic cloves
- 1 tbsp. red wine vinegar
- 3 tbsp. olive oil
- ¼ C. lemon juice
- 4 skin-on, bone-in chicken thighs

How it's made:

- Dry chicken with paper towels.
- Mix salt, parsley, oregano, basil, garlic, vinegar, 2 tbsp olive oil, and lemon juice in a shallow dish. Place chicken in marinade mixture for 60 minutes.
- Ensure oven is preheated to 425 degrees.
- Warm remaining olive oil and sear chicken on all sides until browned.
- Arrange chicken and veggies on a plate. Drizzle with remaining marinade and toss gently.
- Cover with foil and bake 35 minutes till potatoes are softened.

- Then, remove foil and cook 5-10 more minutes till potatoes and chicken become slightly crisp.
  Serve garnished with lemon slices and olives.

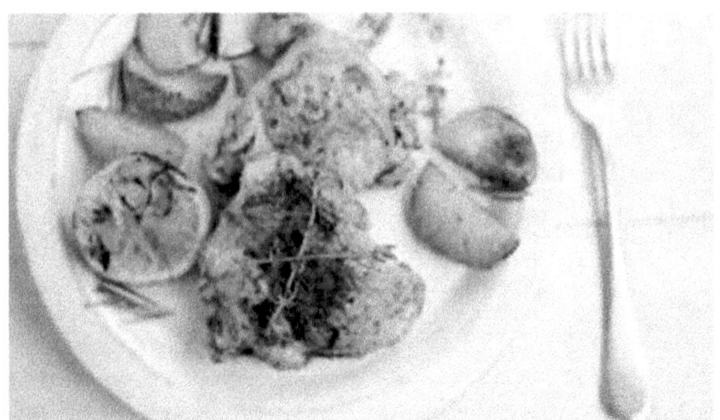

Olive Oil Pasta

What's in it:

- Zest of 1 lemon
- 10-15 basil leaves
- ¼ C. crumbled feta cheese
- ¼ C. pitted/halved olives
- 6 ounces drained artichoke hearts
- 1 tsp. pepper
- 3 chopped scallions
- 12 ounces halved grape tomatoes
- 1 C. chopped parsley
- Salt
- 4 crushed garlic cloves
- ½ C. extra virgin olive oil
- 1 pound spaghetti noodles
- Crushed red pepper flakes

How it's made:

- Cook spaghetti until al dente.
- Warm olive oil and sauté garlic with a couple pinches of salt, cooking 10 seconds.
- Mix in scallions, tomatoes, and parsley. Cover and cook 1 minute.
- Drain water from pasta and pour back into the pot. Pour warmed olive mixture over noodles and toss well. Add pepper and toss again.
- Stir in remaining recipe components and toss well.
- Serve topped with feta and basil.

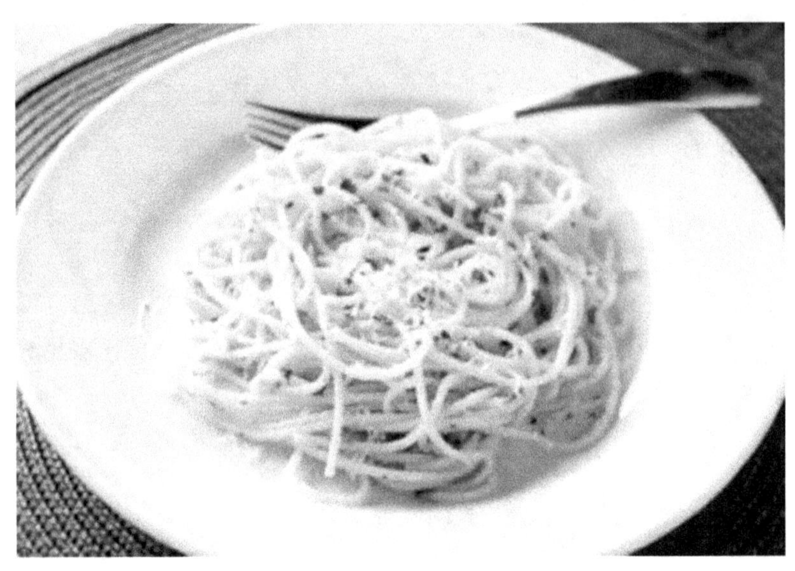

One-Pan Pesto Chicken

What's in it:

- 1 C. uncooked tortellini
- 1 C. cherry tomatoes
- ¼ C. basil pesto
- 1 pound asparagus
- 1/3 C. sun-dried tomatoes
- 1 pound boneless skinless chicken thighs
- 2 tbsp. olive oil

How it's made:

- Warm up olive oil and add thighs, searing on all sides. While searing, add half of tomatoes and season with salt. Cook 5-10 minutes till chicken is cooked thoroughly.
- Take out sun-dried tomatoes and chicken, but leave oil in a pan. Place asparagus in the pan, season with salt and remaining tomatoes and cook 5-10 minutes till asparagus is cooked. Place on serving platter.
- Cook tortellini and drain.
- Place chicken in a pan with pesto, heat 1-2 minutes.
- Take off heat and add cherry tomatoes and tortellini to chicken and pesto.

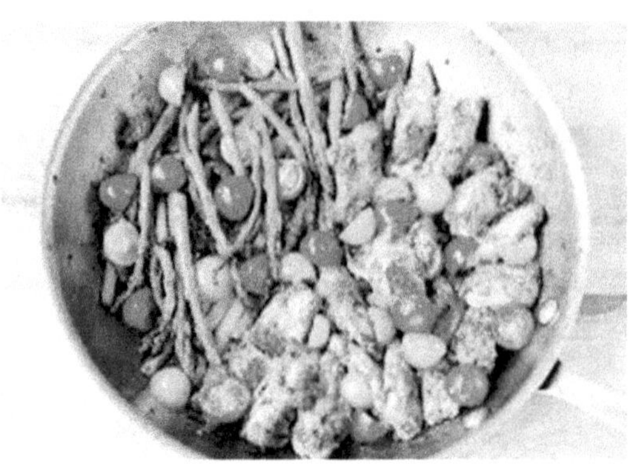

Greek Burgers with Spinach, Feta, and Sun-Dried Tomatoes

What's in it:

Patties:

- ½ tsp. salt
- 1 egg
- 1/3 C. chopped sun-dried tomatoes
- 2 ounces crumbled feta cheese
- 5 ounces chopped baby spinach leaves
- 1 pound ground beef

Toppings and Buns:

- ¼ C. tzatziki sauce
- 1 sliced shallot
- 1 sliced tomato
- 1-ounce spinach leaves
- 4 whole wheat sandwich buns

How it's made:

- Mix all of the patty components together till combined. Form mixture into 4 hamburger patties. Chill 1 hour.
- Heat a pan, drizzling buns with olive oil and placing face down. Cook 1-2 minutes to crisp.
- Turn up the heat and add more oil to the pan. Then add patties, cooking till meat is cooked thoroughly.
- Put burgers together with toppings.

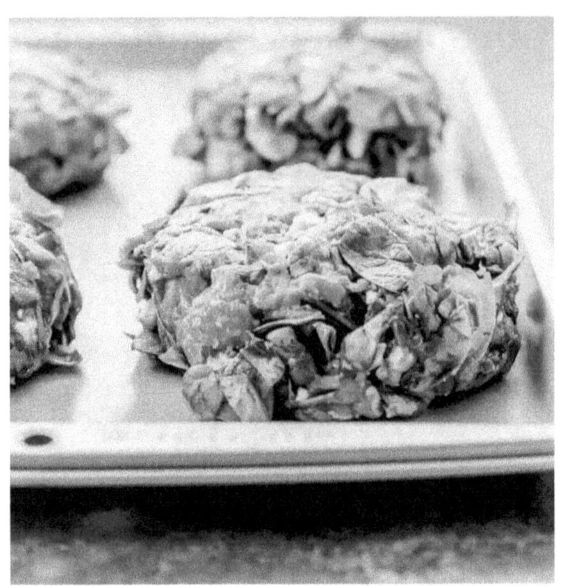

One-Pan Mediterranean Chicken with Roasted Red Pepper Sauce

What's in it:

- 2 tbsp. crumbled feta cheese
- 1 C. heavy cream
- ¼ tsp. pepper
- ½ tsp. salt
- 3 tsp. minced garlic
- 4 tbsp. oil
- 2 tsp. Italian seasoning
- 2/3 C. chopped roasted red peppers
- 4-6 boneless skinless chicken thighs
- Thinly sliced basil

How it's made:

- Mix pepper, salt, garlic, oil, 1 tsp. Italian seasoning, and roasted red peppers to a food processor. Pulse till smooth.
- Grease a pan. Season chicken with remaining Italian seasoning. Cook 6-8 minutes till cooked on all sides thoroughly. Put on a plate to keep warm.
- Pour red pepper mixture into the pan, heating 2-3 minutes. Pour heavy cream in, mixing until creamy.
- Place chicken into mixture and coat meat.
- Garnish with basil and feta cheese.

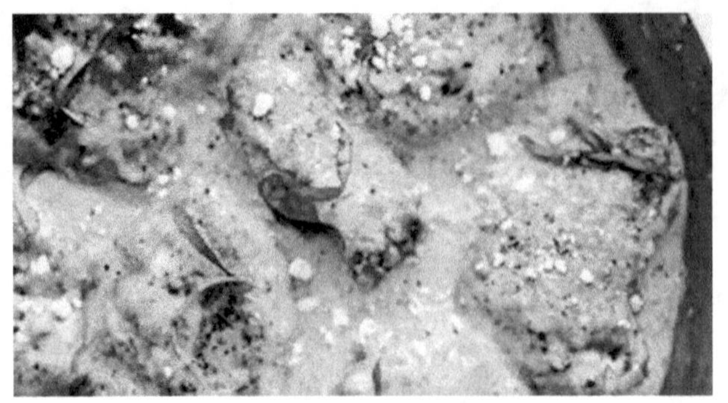

Meatball Gyros Sandwich

What's in it:
- 1 tbsp. chopped parsley
- ½ C. diced red onion
- 1 C. diced tomatoes
- 1 C. diced cucumbers
- ¼ tsp. pepper
- ½ tsp. salt
- ½ tsp. cumin
- 1 tbsp. minced garlic
- 2 tbsp. chopped parsley
- 1 egg
- ¼ C. Italian breadcrumbs
- 1 pound ground chuck
- 1 tbsp. lemon juice
- ¼ tsp. pepper
- ½ tsp. salt
- 1 tbsp. dill
- 1 tsp. extra virgin olive oil
- 1 tsp. minced garlic
- ¼ C. grated cucumber
- 1 C. Greek yogurt
- Pepper and salt
- 4 flatbreads

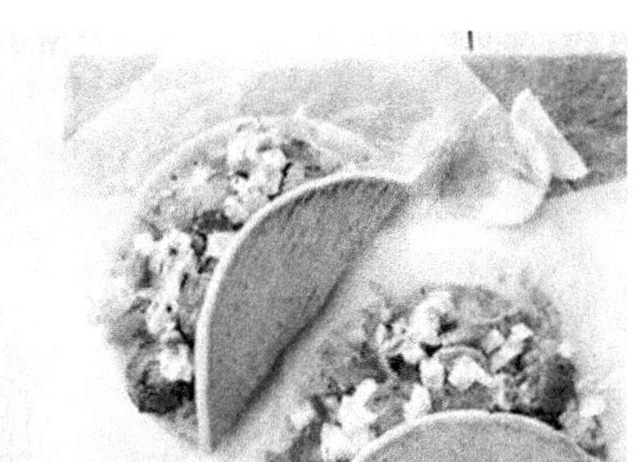

How it's made:
- Mix Greek yogurt, ¼ tsp. pepper, ½ tsp. salt, 1 tbsp. dill, 1 tsp. olive oil, and 1 tsp. garlic. Toss mixture with grated cucumber. Then stir in 1 tbsp. lemon juice and combine well. Chill until ready to eat.
- Ensure oven is preheated to 425 degrees.

- Mix ¼ tsp. pepper, ½ tsp. salt, ½ tsp. cumin, 1 tbsp. garlic, 2 tbsp. parsley, 1 egg, ¼ cup breadcrumbs, and ground chuck till combined.
- Make meatballs out of meat mixture.
- Grease a tray and arrange meatballs upon the tray. Bake 10-15 minutes till cooked.
- Combine parsley, ½ cup red onion, 1 cup tomatoes, and 1 cup cucumbers together and season with pepper and salt.
- Take out meatballs and allow a few minutes to rest.
- To assemble sandwiches, place 4 meatballs in center of flatbread. Pour a liberal amount of sauce onto meatballs and top with cucumber and tomato salad. Wrap and devour!

Tomato Basil Artichoke Baked Chicken

What's in it:

- 8 ounces sliced mozzarella cheese
- ¼ C. parmesan cheese
- 2 minced garlic cloves
- 1 chopped Roma tomato
- 7 chopped basil leaves
- 7 drained artichoke hearts
- 1 tbsp. butter
- Italian seasoning
- Salt
- 4 chicken breasts, cut in half horizontally

How it's made:

- Ensure oven is preheated to 375 degrees. Grease a baking pan.
- Season chicken with Italian seasoning and salt. Place onto the pan and bake 15 minutes.
- Take out of the oven.
- Mix parmesan, garlic, tomato, basil, and artichoke hearts together.
- Spoon mixture onto chicken along with mozzarella cheese.
- Broil 15-20 minutes.
- Eat as is or along with rice and/or spinach. Enjoy!

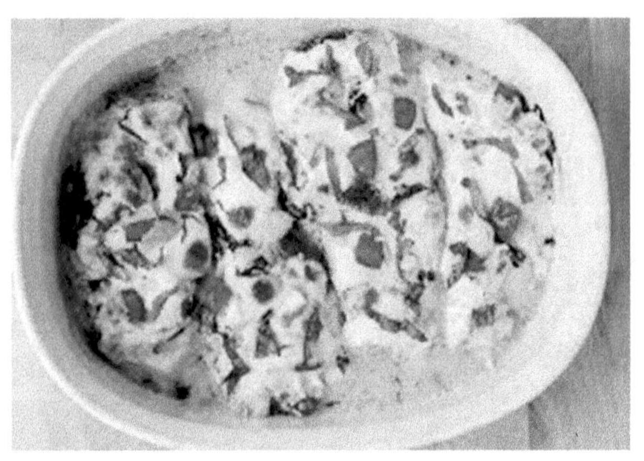

Cucumber Dill Salmon

What's in it:

- ¼ C. + 2-3 tbsp. skim milk
- 2 tbsp. minced dill
- 4 ounces light cream cheese
- 1/3 C. chopped cucumber
- 1 lemon, sliced into wedges
- Pepper and salt
- 3-4 salmon fillets
- Olive oil

How it's made:

- Ensure oven is preheated to 400 degrees. Drizzle olive oil on fish and season with pepper and salt. Place in a skillet.
- Sear salmon on both sides 6-8 minutes, squeezing lemon juice over fish.
- Take fish out of the pan, and add cream cheese and milk. Season with pepper and salt and combine well.
- Take off heat and mix in cucumber and dill, mixing sauce until creamy.
- Sere salmon with dill sauce spooned over fish, with a nice garnish of dill and a lemon wedge. Enjoy!

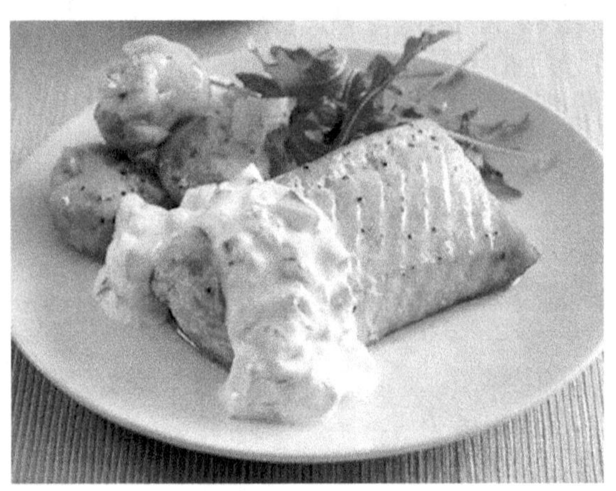

Spiced Lentils and Rice

What's in it:

Lentils and Rice:
- ¼ C. raisins
- ¼ C. pine nuts
- 4 tbsp. chopped cilantro
- ¼ tsp. pepper
- 1 tsp. salt
- 2 tbsp. olive oil
- 1 tsp. coriander
- 1 tsp. cumin
- ½ tsp. allspice
- ½ tsp. chili flakes
- 4 sliced cloves garlic
- 1 C. brown lentils
- 1 C. long grain rice

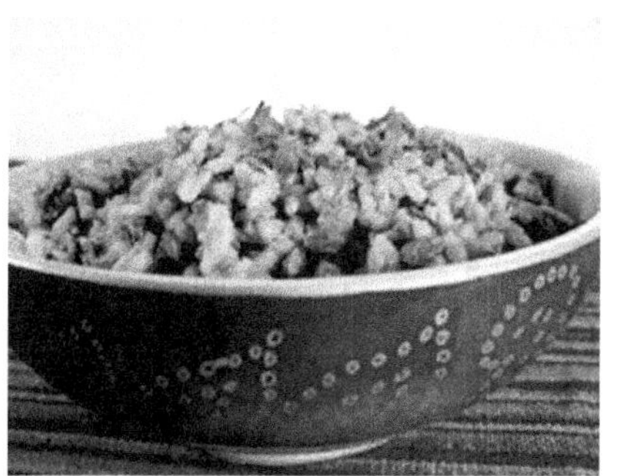

Fried Onion Garnish:
- 3 sliced shallots
- 2 tbsp. all-purpose flour
- Pepper and salt

How it's made:
- Wash lentils in cold water. Pour into a pot with a tsp of salt and 4 cups of water. Heat to boiling, then turn down heat and simmer 17-20 minutes until tender. Drain and put to the side.
- To make fried onions, heat oil and mix ¼ tsp salt along with ½ tsp. pepper. Dredge onions in flour, then add to pan until crispy. Set on a plate lined with paper towels.

- Warm up fresh oil and sauté remaining shallot until tender. Then add in garlic and sauté 30 seconds.
- Pour in rice, toasting with spices for 2 minutes.
- Then stir in cooked lentils, ½ tsp salt and 2 cups of water, adjusting salt as needed to achieve desired taste.
- Heat mixture to boiling, then turn down heat and simmer 10-12 minutes till rice is fully cooked.
- Fold in raisin, pine nuts, and cilantro.
- Serve warm with chutney or yogurt!

One-Pan Salmon with Corn, Zucchini, and Tomatoes

What's in it:

- 2 pounds salmon fillet
- 2 C. halved cherry tomatoes
- 2-3 C. corn
- 3 C. chopped zucchini
- Pepper
- ½ tsp. salt
- 2 tsp. minced garlic
- 2 tsp. oregano
- 2 tbsp. lemon juice
- 1/3 C. olive oil

How it's made:

- Ensure oven is preheated to 400 degrees. With foil, line a tray and grease with cooking spray.
- Whisk pepper, salt, garlic, oregano, lemon juice, and olive oil together.
- Toss zucchini in 2 tbsp of lemon mixture. Spread coated zucchini onto the tray. Roast for 15 minutes.
- Toss tomatoes and corn with 2 tbsp. of lemon mixture.
  Take the pan from oven and add coated tomatoes and corn to zucchini.
- Push veggies to side of the tray and add salmon fillets to pan. Brush with lemon sauce.
- Roast 10 minutes. Remove from oven and toss gently. Then broil 3 minutes to brown salmon.

- Serve drizzled with remaining lemon sauce. Enjoy!

Dessert Recipes

Baklava Cigars

What's in it:
Syrup:
- ½ vanilla bean
- ¼ C. maple syrup
- ¾ C. fresh orange juice

Baklava Cigars:
- 1 tbsp. chopped shelled pistachios
- 2 tbsp. olive oil
- 3 vegan pastry sheets
- ¼ C. + 1 tbsp. maple syrup
- 1/8 tsp. fine sea salt
- 1 ½ tsp. cinnamon
- Zest of 2 oranges
- Zest of 1 lemon
- 1 C. walnuts
- 1 C. almonds

How it's made:
- In a strainer, strain scraped the vanilla bean, maple syrup, and orange juice into a pot. Heat pot to boiling, turn down heat and simmer till syrup is able to coat the back of a spoon. Put to the side to cool down.
- In a food processor, grind nuts till coarse.
- Mix ground nuts with orange and lemon zest, salt, and cinnamon.
- Add zest mixture to maple syrup mixture, incorporating well.
- Grease a tray with olive oil. Have 2 wet kitchen towels at your disposal.
- Open pastry sheets. Remove one sheet and place a towel over other to keep them from drying out.

- Cut the sheet in half, put one half directly in front, the other perpendicular to you.
- Brush pastry lightly with oil. Spoon 2 tbsp. of filling into a sheet. Mold filling into a cigar shape, and roll pastry around filling.
- Put rolls, seam face down, onto the tray.
  Repeat this with remaining ingredients.
- Ensure oven is preheated to 350 degrees.
- Brush tops of cigars with oil. Bake 25 minutes till gold.
- Brush cigars with cooled down syrup and sprinkle with pistachios. Serve!

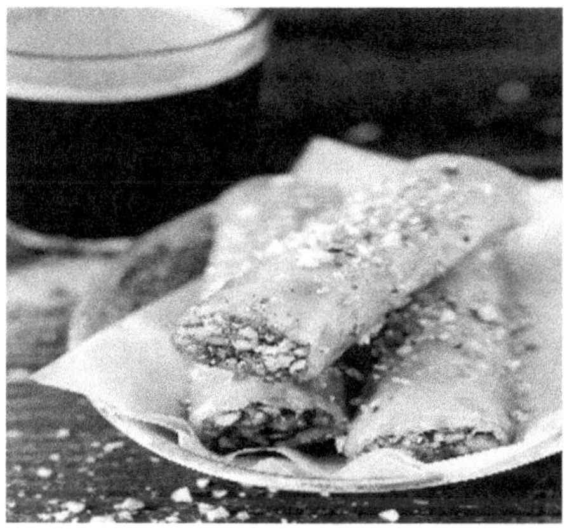

Vanilla Baked Pears

What's in it:

- 1 tsp. vanilla extract
- ¼ tsp. cinnamon
- ½ C. pure maple syrup
- 4 Anjou pears

How it's made:

- Ensure oven is preheated to 375 degrees. With parchment paper, line a tray.
- Slice pears in half. Remove core of pears with a melon baller.
- Place pears facing upwards onto the tray. Sprinkle with cinnamon.
- Mix vanilla extract and maple syrup together. Drizzle over pears, reserving 2 tbsp. for later.
- Bake 25 minutes till softened and golden.
- Drizzle with remaining syrup mixture.

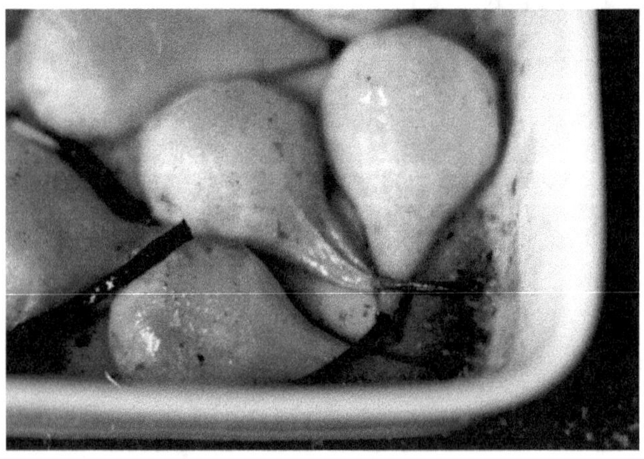

Apple Cake

What's in it:

- 3 tsp. baking powder
- ¼ C. + 2 tbsp. low-fat milk
- 1 C. sifted all-purpose flour
- Pinch of salt
- Zest of 1 lemon
- 1/3 C. + 1 tbsp. light brown sugar
- 2 eggs
- 1 ½ pounds Granny Smith apples

How it's made:

- Ensure oven is preheated to 350 degrees. Flour and grease a dish.
- Peel, core and thinly cut apples.
- Mix salt, lemon zest, sugar, and eggs together in a mixer till creamy. Then beat in milk, baking powder, and flour.
- Mix 2/3 of apples into the batter with a spoon.
- Pour batter into dish.
- Arrange remaining apple slices over batter and sprinkle with brown sugar.
- Bake 35 minutes.
- Dust with powdered sugar before serving if you desire.

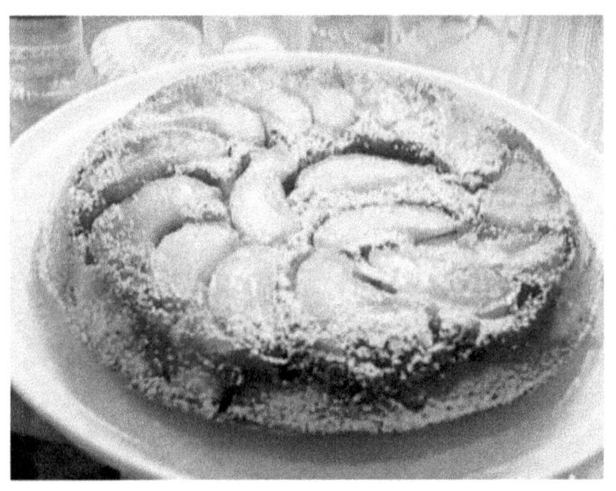

Almond Coconut Semolina Cake

What's in it:

- ¼ C. shaved almonds
- ¼ C. sweetened shredded coconut
- 1 tsp. baking powder
- 1/3 C. milk
- 1 C. fine semolina
- 1 C. coarse semolina
- 1 C. plain yogurt
- 1 C. sugar
- ½ C. + 2 tbsp. unsalted butter

Cinnamon Syrup:

- ¼ tsp. lemon juice
- 1 cinnamon stick
- 1 ¾ C. water
- 1 ½ C. sugar

How it's made:

- Ensure oven is preheated to 350 degrees. Grease a baking dish.
- Melt butter in the microwave.
- Combine yogurt and sugar together. Then add both semolina, milk, and baking powder. Stir in melted butter till well incorporated.
- Pour batter into prepared dish. Bake 40-45 minutes.
- As cake bakes, combine cinnamon stick, water, and sugar in a pan. Heat to boiling, stirring until sugar dissolves. Turn down heat and simmer a few minutes.

Take off heat and mix in lemon juice. Allow to totally cool, and discard cinnamon stick.

- Take the cake from oven and top with syrup. Let cool an hour before serving.
- When ready to devour, sprinkle cake with coconut and almonds.

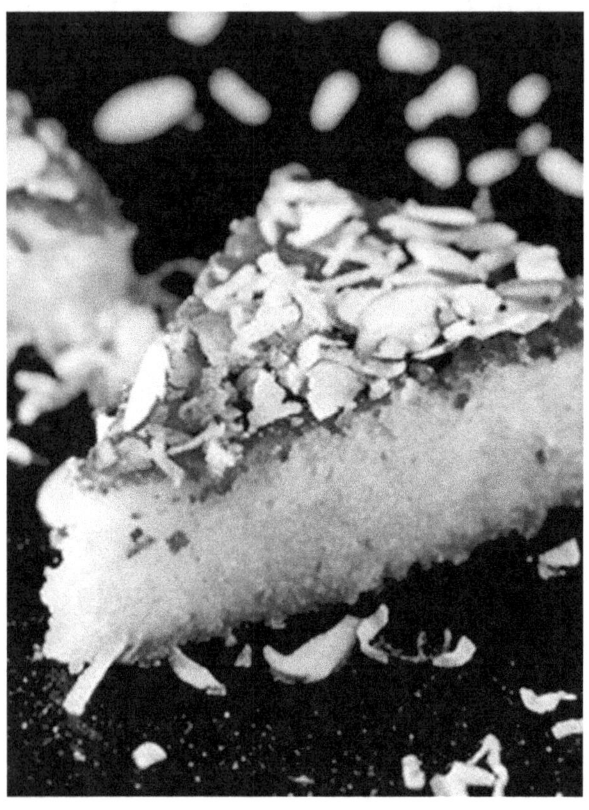

Berry Clafoutis

What's in it:

- Zest of ½ a lemon
- 6 ounces blueberries
- 6 ounces blackberries
- 1 tbsp. granulated sweetener of choice
- 1 tsp. butter
- 1 ½ tsp. vanilla extract
- 1 C. half and half
- 3 eggs
- Pinch of salt
- 1 C. powdered sweetener of choice
- ½ tsp. baking powder
- 1/3 C. all-purpose flour

How it's made:

- Ensure oven is preheated to 375 degrees. Grease a pan with butter.
- Mix powdered sweeteners, baking powder, and flour together.
- In another bowl, beat vanilla extract, half and half, and eggs together with an electric mixer will smooth.
- Combine wet and dry mixture together with mixer until a nice and smooth batter is created. Stir in lemon zest.
- Dust surface of the pan with granulated sweetener and pour mixed berries into the pan. Pour batter over berries.
- Bake 30-35 minutes till puffy and golden.
- To serve, dust with powdered sweetener and eat warm!

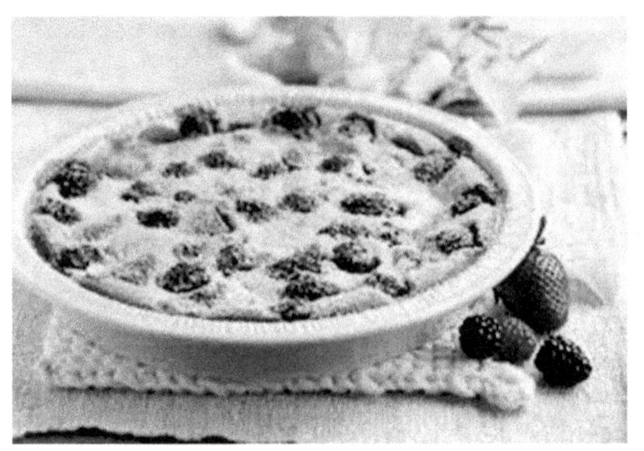

Strawberry and Pistachio Tart

What's in it:

- ¼ C. crushed pistachios
- 18-20 thinly sliced strawberries
- 1 thawed sheet puff pastry
- 3 tbsp honey + more for drizzling
- 6 ounces softened cream cheese

How it's made:

- Ensure oven is preheated to 400 degrees. With parchment paper, line a tray.
- Beat honey and cream cheese together until fluffy.
- Lay out pastry sheet onto the tray. Spread honey mixture on pastry, smoothing gently.
- Spread strawberries onto cream cheese, making sure to leave at least a ½" border. Stack remaining strawberries.
- Fold the edges inward.
- Bake 18-22 minutes till crust is golden and strawberries are caramelized.
- Drizzle tart with additional honey and sprinkle with pistachios.

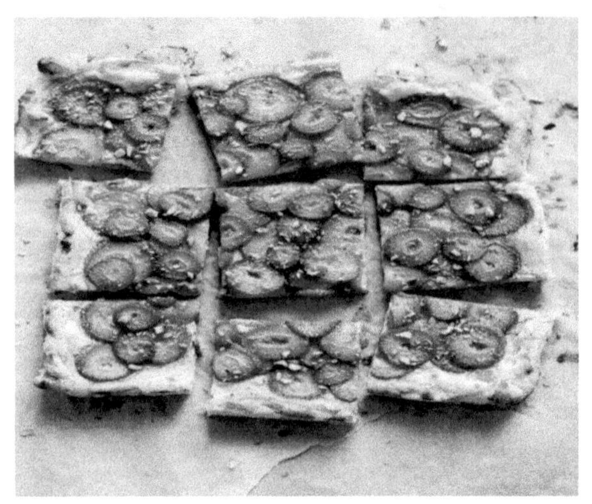

Figs with Mascarpone, Honey, and Pistachios

What's in it:

- ¼ C. toasted/chopped pistachios
- 1-pint fresh figs
- ¾ tsp. vanilla extract
- ½ tsp. lemon zest
- 2 tsp. lemon juice
- 2-3 tbsp. honey
- 2 C. mascarpone

How it's made:

- Combine vanilla extract, lemon zest, lemon juice, honey, and mascarpone together.
- To serve, spoon mascarpone mixture into a bowl. Top with figs, pistachios, and honey.
- Enjoy this easy dessert!

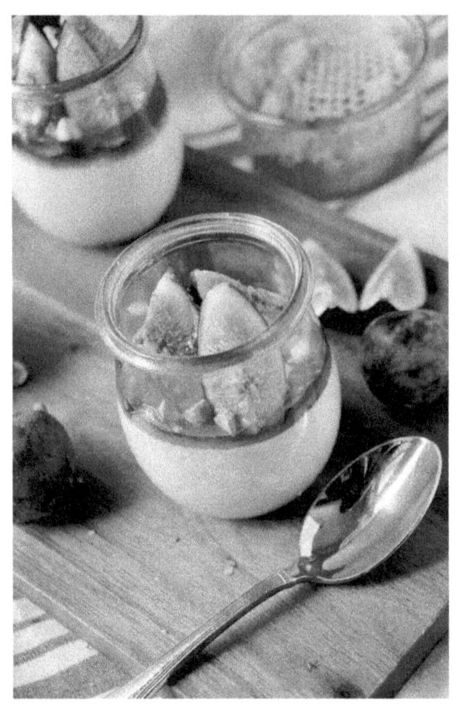

Apple Olive Oil Cake

What's in it:

- 1 tsp. bicarbonate of soda
- 1 tsp. baking powder
- ½ tsp. cinnamon
- 3 eggs
- Zest of 1 lemon
- 2/3 C. sultanas golden
- 2 sweet green apples
- 7 ounces olive oil
- 1 C. fine light brown sugar
- 3 C. flour

How it's made:

- Ensure oven is preheated to 350 degrees. Grease cake pan with butter and dust with flour.
- Soak sultanas 10-15 minutes in warm water.
- Whisk sugar and olive oil together 2 minutes. Then mix in bicarbonate, baking powder, cinnamon, and flour. Fold in lemon zest, apple, and sultanas.
- Pour batter into cake pan.
- Bake 45 minutes.
- Let cool before slicing.

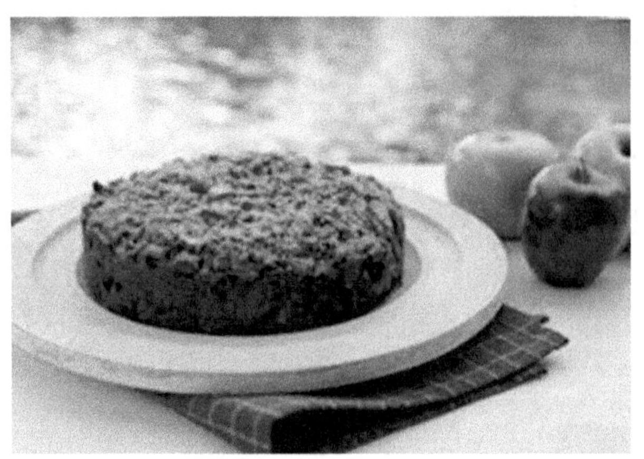

Cinnamon and Spice Sweet Potato Bread

What's in it:

- Pinch of salt
- ½ tsp. ground cloves
- ½ tsp. allspice
- 1 tsp. nutmeg
- 1 tbsp. cinnamon
- 2 tsp. baking soda
- ¼ C. light brown sugar
- 1 ¼ C. granulated sweetener of choice
- 1 ¾ C. all-purpose flour
- 1 tsp. vanilla extract
- ¼ C. Greek yogurt
- ½ C. vegetable oil
- 2 eggs
- 3 tbsp. water
- 1 ½ C. mashed sweet potatoes

How it's made:

- Ensure oven is preheated to 350 degrees. Grease a loaf pan.
- Add 3 tbsp water to chopped sweet potatoes and pop in the microwave. Heat 15-17 minutes till potatoes are tender. Mash with a fork and let cool.
- Add vanilla, yogurt, oil, and eggs to sweet potatoes.
- Combine all dry components together.
- Combine wet and dry mixtures together till well incorporated.
- Pour batter into loaf pan(s).

- Bake 60-70 minutes.
  During last 15 minutes of cooking, take foil and create a tent over bread.
- Let cool 10 minutes.

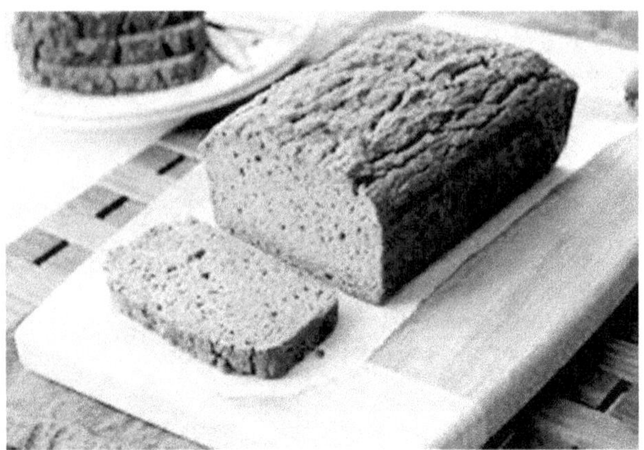

No-Bake Chocolate Nut Protein Cookies

What's in it:

- 2 tbsp. coconut oil
- ½ C. agave
- 1 ½ C. almond butter
- 3 scoops chocolate protein powder
- 3 C. oatmeal

How it's made:

- Mix all recipe components together till well incorporated.
- Create balls from the mixture.
- Place onto a tray lined with parchment paper.
- Chill 1-2 hours and devour!

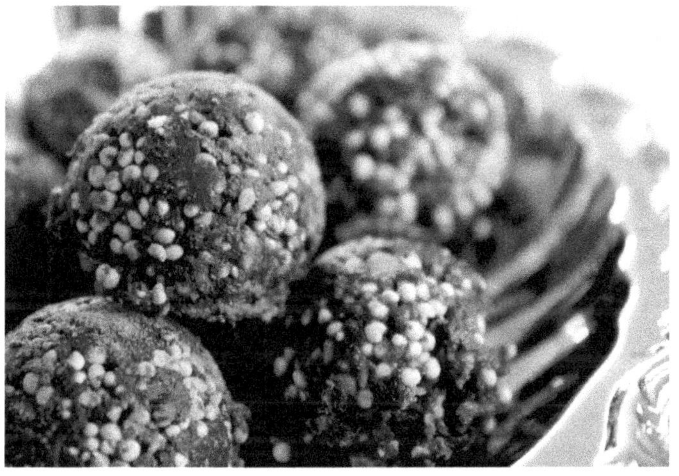

Conclusion

Congratulations! You have now read through the *Mediterranean Diet*!

I hope that getting a taste and premiere look at the Mediterranean diet firsthand has given you just the motivation you need to begin your weight loss journey! I am sure you have fallen in love with at least a few of these recipes in this book, so what are you waiting for?!

It is now your turn to take this valuable cookbook and turn it into a beautiful array of feasts for the family! You are now able to experience the Mediterranean diet up close and personal!

The best thing about this diet is in reality, it isn't necessarily a diet, but a new way of fueling your body. I always like to remind folks that we only get blessed with one body in this lifetime, so why not take care of it the best we can! I want to pat you on the back for making the decision to purchase this book to better your future and to create the *best* version of yourself possible!

It's time to pick out a couple recipes, head to the store, and start making irresistible food that welcome family and friends alike, right from your own kitchen! I hope you see that there is a 'master chef' in you, all you have to do is test out these recipes!

Good luck on your journey through the Mediterranean diet. I hope it brings you not only delicious meals but the ability to shed unwanted pounds as well.

Did you find this cookbook valuable and useful? If so, please take a moment of your time to leave a review on Amazon. It's greatly appreciated! Happy cooking!